COMPLETE GUIDE TO RESPIRATORY CARE IN ATHLETES

Complete Guide to Respiratory Care in Athletes introduces the respiratory system and its function during exercise. It considers the main respiratory conditions affecting athletes and delivers practical advice for the management of respiratory issues in athletic populations.

With contributions from leading international experts, the book discusses fundamental scientific principles and provides pragmatic 'hands-on' clinical guidance to enable practical application. Each chapter includes useful pedagogical features such as case studies and guides for carrying out assessments. The book covers wide a range of topics, including:

- respiratory system function during exercise
- impact of the environment on the upper and lower airways
- asthma related issues in athletes
- allergic rhinitis in athletes
- exercise induced laryngeal obstruction
- exercise induced dysfunctional breathing patterns
- respiratory muscle training
- role of screening for respiratory issues in athletes
- assessing and dealing with respiratory infections in athletes.

This text is key reading for both newly qualified and established medical, scientific and therapy practitioners who are working with athletes with respiratory issues. It is also a valuable resource for students of sports medicine, sports therapy, and sport and exercise science courses.

John W. Dickinson, PhD is Reader within the School of Sport and Exercise Science at the University of Kent, UK. He has over 17 years' experience of helping athletes optimise their airway health, over this time he has seen in excess of 2,000 athletes. His work has influenced policy on the management of athlete respiratory health and assisted practitioners to differentiate between various respiratory problems experienced by athletes. He has worked with elite organisations including British Olympic Association, English Institute of Sport, The Football Association and UK Anti-Doping. He has also featured in multiple media stories explaining respiratory issues faced by athletes.

James H. Hull, PhD, FRCP, FACSM is a consultant respiratory physician at the Royal Brompton Hospital, London, UK and Hon. Senior Lecturer, Imperial College London. He has a specialist clinical and research interest in helping athletic individuals with unexplained breathlessness, wheeze and cough. He has worked with a number of elite and professional sporting organisations to optimise athlete respiratory care, including British Swimming, the English Institute of Sport, UK Anti-doping and the International Olympic Committee.

COMPLETE GUIDE TO RESPIRATORY CARE IN ATHLETES

Edited by John W. Dickinson and James H. Hull

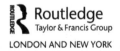
Routledge
Taylor & Francis Group

LONDON AND NEW YORK

First published 2020
by Routledge
2 Park Square, Milton Park, Abingdon, Oxon OX14 4RN

and by Routledge
52 Vanderbilt Avenue, New York, NY 10017

Routledge is an imprint of the Taylor & Francis Group, an informa business

British Library Cataloguing-in-Publication Data
A catalogue record for this book is available from the British Library

Library of Congress Cataloging-in-Publication Data
Names: Dickinson, John (John W.), editor.
Title: Complete guide to respiratory care in athletes / edited by John Dickinson and James Hull.
Description: Milton Park, Abingdon, Oxon ; New York, NY : Routledge, 2020. | Includes bibliographical references and index.
Identifiers: LCCN 2020004701 (print) | LCCN 2020004702 (ebook) | ISBN 9781138588349 (hardback) | ISBN 9781138588356 (paperback) | ISBN 9780429492341 (ebook)
Subjects: LCSH: Respiratory organs--Physiology. | Sports--Physiological aspects.
Classification: LCC RC1236.R47 C66 2020 (print) | LCC RC1236.R47 (ebook) | DDC 616.2002/4796--dc23
LC record available at https://lccn.loc.gov/2020004701
LC ebook record available at https://lccn.loc.gov/2020004702

ISBN: 978-1-138-58834-9 (hbk)
ISBN: 978-1-138-58835-6 (pbk)
ISBN: 978-0-429-49234-1 (ebk)

Typeset in Bembo
by Taylor & Francis Books

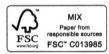

MIX
Paper from
responsible sources
FSC
www.fsc.org   FSC™ C013985

Printed in the United Kingdom
by Henry Ling Limited

CONTENTS

FIGURES

TABLES

CONTRIBUTORS

Emily Adamic is a graduate student in the Department of Kinesiology at Indiana University, Bloomington, Indiana, USA. In addition to studying the cardio-pulmonary limitations to exercise performance and the role of non-pharmacological interventions to respiratory health in athletes, her main research focus is integrative exercise physiology, specifically central nervous system control of exercise intensity, and the role of sensory afferent information in exercise-induced fatigue. She has also worked in an applied sport science environment, working as a sport physiologist part of an integrated support team to test and monitor high-level athletes for the ultimate goal of athletic performance.

Bruno Archiza, PhD received his Bachelor's degree in Physical Therapy from the Federal University of São Carlos (Brazil) in 2013. In 2014, he started his Master's in Physical Therapy at the same institution, which later that year was transferred to a PhD through the grant of a scholarship. In 2016, he was received as an international student at the University of British Columbia (Canada) under the mentorship of Dr Bill Sheel. In 2018 and back to Brazil, Bruno completed his PhD under the mentorship of Dr Audrey Borghi-Silva. Working once more alongside Dr Sheel, Bruno is currently a postdoctoral fellow in the School of Kinesiology at the University of British Columbia. His research focuses on diaphragmatic fatigue and sex-based differences.

Anna Boniface, MCSP worked as a specialist respiratory physiotherapist in the National Health Service (UK) in acute respiratory medicine before moving into chronic respiratory disease management at St Mary's Hospital, Paddington and Berkshire Health Care NHS Trust. Through these roles, Anna became interested in Breathing Pattern Disorders. From being immersed in elite endurance sport as an athlete, Anna became more interested in breathing pattern disorders within the athletic population. Anna now works as a specialist musculoskeletal physiotherapist at Flint

House Police Rehabilitation Centre, providing intensive physiotherapy to injured police officers. With the combination of musculoskeletal and respiratory physiotherapy, Anna treats athletes with breathing pattern disorders privately in the Reading area.

Matteo Bonini, MD is an Assistant Professor at the Department of Cardiothoracic Sciences of the Catholic University of Rome and Honorary Clinical Senior Lecturer at the National Heart and Lung Institute of the Imperial College London. He is a Board Certified in Sports Medicine, PhD in 'Allergy and Respiratory Diseases'. He is also a 'Marie-Curie' and 'ERS Long-Term' Fellowship recipient. He is licensed as a Full Professor in 'Internal Medicine' and 'Exercise and Sports Medicine' and as Associate Professor in 'Cardiovascular and Respiratory Diseases' by the Italian Ministry of University and Research.

John Brannan, MD is the Scientific Director, Department of Respiratory and Sleep Medicine at the John Hunter Hospital, NSW Australia. He is a specialist in bronchial challenge testing for the assessment of asthma and exercise-induced bronchoconstriction. Early in his academic career, he worked with Drs Anderson and Daviskas on some of the emerging studies on the investigation of dry powders for bronchial provocation. He was an integral member of the research team that led the mannitol test to be the first registered bronchial provocation test in Australia. Dr Brannan has published 66 papers in peer-reviewed journals and four book chapters. He has been an invited speaker to both national and international meetings.

Hege Havstad Clemm, MD, PhD, is currently working as a Head Consultant at Department of Pediatrics, Haukeland University Hospital, Bergen, Norway and as an Associate Professor at Department of Clinical Science, University of Bergen, Norway. She is a Pediatric Pulmonologist and a Sports Physician, and is part of the National Olympic Committee of Western Norway. Presently she is the main physician for the Norwegian Olympic candidates in triathlon. Based on EILO-research done by the Bergen EILO-group since 1997, she established an outpatient clinic at Haukeland University Hospital in 2010, a cooperation between the Head and Neck Surgery Department and the Pediatric Department, serving patients with EILO from all Norway. In 2013 she established an EILO-registry based on this clinic. She is running the EILO-register and the EILO/ILO-research group in Bergen, Norway. She is also respiratory and medical advisor to the anti-doping organisation in Norway, board member of Norwegian Pediatric Pulmonology Association and board member of Western Norway Sports Medicine Association. She is an associate editor to the Norwegian Journal of Sports Medicine and was the head of the Annual Norwegian Congress of Sports Medicine, held in Bergen, Norway in 2018.

Glen Davison, PhD attained his first degree in Sport and Exercise Sciences at Sheffield Hallam University in 2001 and MSc in Exercise Physiology in September 2002. He commenced his PhD on 'Nutrition and Exercise Immunology' in October 2002 at Loughborough University. While at Loughborough Glen also worked as a Teaching Assistant in Exercise Physiology. He worked as a lecturer in Sports Nutrition and

Exercise Physiology at Aberystwyth University for just over 5 years before joining the SSES, University of Kent, in September 2011. Dr Davison is also a BASES Accredited sport and exercise scientist (Physiology) and a Chartered Scientist (CSci). He has worked with amateur, elite and professional athletes from a range of sports, including Football, Rugby, Hockey, Athletics, Triathlon and Cycling. His current interests include: Nutrition and Exercise Immunology; Interval training; Sport & Exercise Science support of athletes (i.e. maintaining optimal health and performance) in sports including Football, Rugby, Hockey, Athletics, Endurance/LD running, Triathlon and Cycling; Exercise Immunology in people with Diabetes. Exercise and Immune function in people with Chronic Obstructive Pulmonary Disease (COPD); Exercise in people with Parkinson's Disease.

John W. Dickinson PhD is Reader within the School of Sport and Exercise Science at the University of Kent, UK. He has over 17 years' experience of helping athletes optimise their airway health, over this time he has seen in excess of 2,000 athletes. His work has influenced policy on the management of athlete respiratory health, helping practitioners differentiate between various respiratory problems experienced by athletes.

Jon Greenwell MD, has worked in high-performance sport for the past 10 years, predominately in endurance sport with swimmers, cyclists and triathletes. He currently works at the English Institute for Sport with British Triathlon. He has been an advocate for screening for respiratory disorders for many years to optimise health and minimise the substantial burden of respiratory illness in sports people

James H. Hull PhD, FRCP, FACSM is a consultant respiratory physician at the Royal Brompton Hospital, London, UK and Hon. Senior Lecturer, Imperial College London. He has a specialist clinical and research interest in helping athletic individuals with unexplained breathlessness, wheeze and cough. He has worked with a number of elite and professional sporting organisations, to optimise athlete respiratory care, including British Swimming, the English Institute of Sport, UK Anti-doping and the International Olympic Committee.

Michael Johnson, PhD, is a Senior Lecturer and member of the Exercise and Health Research Group in the Department of Sport Science at Nottingham Trent University, UK. Dr Johnson's research interests include the effects of dietary intervention, including prebiotics, on exercise-induced asthma, the responses and limitations of the pulmonary system during exercise, and the role of peripheral and central fatigue in limiting exercise tolerance. Dr Johnson has written scientific papers on these topics, which have been published in peer reviewed scientific journals. He is a reviewer for several professional journals, a member of the European Respiratory Society, and a Fellow of the Higher Education Academy. Dr Johnson was awarded his PhD in Exercise Physiology from Nottingham Trent University in 2005, where he studied the responses of the respiratory muscles to training and endurance exercise.

Pascale Kippelen, PhD is a Senior Lecturer in Exercise & Respiratory Physiology at Brunel University London. After completing undergraduate (BSc) and post-graduate studies (MSc and PhD) in Sport & Exercise Sciences in France, she joined Dr Sandra D Anderson at the Dept. of Respiratory Medicine, Royal Prince Alfred Hospital, Sydney (Australia) to carry on post-doctoral training. There, she investigated the pathophysiology of exercise-induced bronchoconstriction in athletes, and took part to phase III of the clinical trial for Aridol/Osmohale, which is a bronchial provocation test aimed at diagnosing asthma patients and managing the condition. Dr Kippelen has published extensively in the field of exercise-induced broncho-constriction, particularly demonstrating the contribution of airway epithelial injury to the pathogenesis of exercise-induced bronchoconstriction in elite athletes. She regularly advises high-profile sporting organisations (such as the International Olympic Committee – Medical Commission and UK-Anti Doping) on issues relating to treatment of asthma/exercise-induced bronchoconstriction in elite sport.

Michael Koehle, MD, PhD is a Professor and Director of Sport & Exercise Medicine at the University of British Columbia. He obtained his MD from the University of Toronto and his PhD in Exercise Physiology from the University of British Columbia. His research program combines exercise and environmental physiology ranging from basic mechanistic research to clinical field studies in remote environments and applied research for high-performance sport. Key research areas include high altitude medicine and physiology, and the physiology of exercise in polluted air. As a physiologist, he runs the Environmental Physiology Laboratory in the School of Kinesiology at the University of British Columbia, and works closely with the Canadian Sport Institute Pacific in applied sport science research. His work has been funded by Own The Podium, the Canadian Sport Institute, Health Canada, the World Anti-Doping Agency and the Natural Science and Engineering Research Council. He practices Sport and Exercise Medicine at the Allan McGavin Sport Medicine Centre. As a physician, he works with a number of elite and professional athletes, in both summer and winter sports.

Timothy Mickleborough, PhD is a professor in the Department of Kinesiology at Indiana University, Bloomington, Indiana, USA. His main research focus is integrative (whole-body) human exercise physiology; in particular the interactions between the respiratory and cardiovascular systems in health and disease, with emphasis on intervention studies in healthy trained/untrained individuals, the pathophysiology of respiratory disorders in athletes such as asthma and expiratory flow limitation, and the potential cardiorespiratory limitations to exercise tolerance and performance. Research related to respiratory muscle function is directed at the respiratory system determinants of fatigue in health and disease and encompasses respiratory and circulatory mechanics, neurophysiology, muscle physiology, perception of effort and biochemistry.

Tod Olin, MD is a pulmonologist and director of the Exercise Breathing Center at National Jewish Health. He has published in the area of paediatric airways disease, as well as in the area of high-performance exercise limitation. He is specifically interested in helping children and adults exercise safely and comfortably, whether sick or well, fit or obese, toddlers or Olympic-level athletes. Most recently, he has invented two novel therapies for exercise-induced laryngeal obstruction (also known as vocal cord dysfunction), a condition for which Dr Olin is considered a global leader. The first of these interventions, a procedure known as therapeutic laryngoscopy during exercise, was published in the fall of 2016. The second innovation, a series of breathing techniques known as the Olin EILOBI breathing techniques, was published in 2017. Dr Olin also sees the value in working with sporting bodies to promote population health and works with multiple local and national sporting bodies.

Oliver Price, PhD is a Senior Lecturer in Exercise and Respiratory Physiology at Leeds Beckett University, UK. Oliver was awarded a BSc (Hons.) in Sport and Exercise Science (2009) and Masters of Research in Exercise Physiology (2010) from Nottingham Trent University. Following graduation, Oliver received training in respiratory medicine, exercise testing and pulmonary rehabilitation working as a clinical physiologist in the Department of Specialist Medicine – University Hospital Southampton NHS Trust. Oliver completed a PhD in exercise and respiratory physiology between 2011 and 2014 (Northumbria University at Newcastle). Oliver's programme of research evaluated the accuracy of diagnostic methods employed to detect airway dysfunction in athletes and assessed the dissociation between self-report respiratory symptoms and objective physiological testing. Oliver completed post-doctoral research training in cardiovascular physiology at the International Centre for Circulatory Health (ICCH) – Imperial College London – National Heart and Lung Institute (NHLI), before joining Leeds Beckett University in 2015. Oliver is a European Respiratory Society (ERS) Fellowship recipient, ERS Task Force Member (exercise and asthma management), and an elected board member for the European Academy of Allergy and Clinical Immunology (EAACI) – Allergy, Asthma and Sport Working Group. Oliver also leads Sport Asthma – an unexplained exertional breathlessness service.

Guy Scadding, MD is a consultant allergist at the Royal Brompton and Harefield NHS Trust, London and an Honorary Senior Clinical Lecturer at Imperial College. His clinical interests include rhinitis and rhinosinusitis, anaphylaxis, food and drug allergy. He completed a PhD in 2016 on nasal allergen provocation, local biomarkers in nasal fluid and the effects of allergen immunotherapy.

Emil Schwartz Walsted, MD, PhD is Medical doctor and PhD with a special interest in dyspnoea and the larynx and a particular fondness for respiratory physiology, translational research and frontier technology. Besides clinical work, he is an active researcher focusing on exercise-induced laryngeal obstruction (EILO) and vocal cord dysfunction (VCD) – conditions that can mimic asthma and cause breathlessness and wheeze. He is based in Copenhagen at Bispebjerg Hospital and is Hon. Clinical Researcher at Royal Brompton Hospital, London.

Andrew William Sheel, PhD completed his education at Canadian institutions (University of New Brunswick, University of British Columbia, Canada) followed by postdoctoral training at the University of Wisconsin-Madison. He is currently a Professor in the School of Kinesiology and Adjunct Professor in the Faculty of Medicine at UBC. He has several editorial duties for scientific journals including: Associate Editor for Medicine & Science in Sports and Exercise; Sr Editor for Experimental Physiology and Editorial Board Member for the Journal of Applied Physiology. The objective of his research program is to understand how the human respiratory and cardiovascular systems interact, respond and adapt to physiological stressors such as exercise, hypoxia and disease.

Andrew Simpson, PhD is a Lecturer in Exercise and Respiratory Physiology, in the department for Sport, Health and Exercise Science, at the University of Hull. Andrew was awarded his PhD from Brunel University in 2015, for a thesis investigating the pathophysiology of exercise-induced bronchoconstriction in athletes. This topic complemented his undergraduate qualification in sport and exercise science, and his clinical experience as a respiratory physiologist at Imperial College London. Before taking up his role at Hull, Dr Simpson completed post-doc training at the University of Manchester, investigating the role of health technology in asthma self-management.

Karl P Sylvester, PhD is Head of Joint Respiratory Physiology at both Cambridge University Hospitals and Royal Papworth Hospital NHS Foundation Trusts and Lead Healthcare Scientist at Royal Papworth Hospital NHS Foundation Trust. Other current roles include Secretary of Group 9.1 at the European Respiratory Society, a group which represents respiratory and sleep scientists from across Europe and Professional Clinical Advisor for the European Lung Foundation. He spent 6 years as Honorary Chair of the Association for Respiratory Technology & Physiology (ARTP) and now has roles on many ARTP sub-committees. He co-leads the BTS/ARTP Short Course on Respiratory Physiology. He has over twenty years' experience in the performance and interpretation of simple to complex respiratory physiological investigations with a specialist interest is the performance and interpretation of clinical cardio-pulmonary exercise testing (CPET). He is faculty lead for the ARTP's annual CPET course, faculty member for the University of California, Los Angeles/Cambridge CPET course and has given countless independent lectures on CPET. Dr Sylvester initially joined Cambridge University Hospitals after completing a PhD investigating respiratory complications in patients with sickle cell disease.

Joseph Welch, PhD is a Post-Doctoral Research Fellow at the University of Florida, USA. Joseph received his Bachelor's and Master's degrees in Sport and Exercise Science from the University of Derby (UK). In 2018, Joseph completed his PhD in Kinesiology at the University of British Columbia (Canada) under the mentorship of Dr Bill Sheel. During doctoral training, Joseph examined sex differences in diaphragmatic fatigue, including its influence on sympathetic cardiovascular control and exercise tolerance. Working alongside Dr Gordon Mitchell and Dr Emily Fox, Joseph's current research focuses on the neural control of breathing and therapeutic effects of acute intermittent hypoxia.

Neil Williams, PhD is a Senior Lecturer in Exercise Physiology and Nutrition in the Department of Sport Science at Nottingham Trent University (NTU). He established the research of exercise induced asthma and dietary supplementation at NTU where he completed his PhD. Dr Williams's current research focuses on investigating the role of dietary interventions and the gut microbiota in respiratory health (asthma and upper respiratory symptoms); athlete health and exercise performance. In relation to respiratory health the research primarily focuses on the use of prebiotic interventions to reduce airway inflammation and asthma severity. Neil is also interested in the role of the gut microbiota in exercise performance and athlete health and whether favourable manipulation through diet using pre- and probiotics can have a positive effect for the athlete and recreational exerciser. Dr Williams has published high quality research over the past five years gaining national and international coverage of his work; and has been an invited speaker at scientific meetings worldwide. Previously he has successfully led teams of researchers on projects involving the physiological assessment of the armed forces for the Ministry of Defence and commercial clients in a range of extreme environments.

FOREWORD

If you can't breathe optimally, you can't perform optimally.

Pretty obvious you would think, but of the three body systems contributing most to athletic performance – cardiovascular, respiratory and musculoskeletal – the respiratory system is the least appreciated. This book will go a long way to rectifying that anomaly.

For the first half of my sports medicine career, I was blissfully unaware of the importance of respiratory conditions such as exercise-induced bronchospasm (EIB). Why was that? We were taught at medical school that you diagnosed asthma on the basis of an expiratory wheeze and that exercise frequently brought on the symptoms. Thanks to people like Dr John Dickinson and Dr James Hull, I became aware that EIB can present in a whole variety of ways and is not necessarily associated with a wheeze. Symptoms like cough, chest tightness, fatigue and reduced performance can all be due to EIB, and once we started screening to identify those athletes with bronchoconstriction with exercise, I was shocked to discover how common it was and largely undiagnosed. The effect of initiating appropriate treatment was, on many occasions, dramatic and led to much improved performance.

This book is not just about asthma and EIB though. There are a number of respiratory conditions that can affect athletic performance. I remember the first case of exercise-induced laryngeal obstruction, or as it was then called vocal cord dysfunction, presenting with inspiratory stridor loud enough to be heard on the other side of the pitch. The poor girl had been mis-labelled as asthmatic and not surprisingly failed to respond to treatment. Understanding the cause of the dramatic symptoms was a great relief to the young athlete and her parents.

The effect of the environment on respiratory function was never more obvious that in the lead up to the 2008 Beijing Olympic Games. All of a sudden, respiratory medicine was at the forefront of sports medicine.

And then of course there are respiratory tract infections, both upper and lower, which severely impact on sporting performance and can destroy a lifetime preparation for a major event.

This book will be a valuable addition for the sports physician, team doctor, respiratory physician, general practitioner and exercise scientist – anyone who manages those who exercise. I can think of no better authors for a book of this nature than Dr John Dickinson and Dr James Hull, both vastly experienced and knowledgeable, whose athletes have benefitted from their care for many years. Together with celebrated international colleagues, they have put together the definitive text on respiratory care in athletes. A job well done.

Peter Brukner OAM, MBBS, FACSEP
Sport and Exercise Physician
Professor of Sports Medicine, La Trobe University, Melbourne, Australia
Author, *Brukner & Khan's Clinical Sports Medicine*

PROLOGUE: WHY BOTHER MONITORING AND OPTIMISING BREATHING ISSUES IN ATHLETIC INDIVIDUALS?

John W. Dickinson and James H. Hull

Athlete: *"When I perform high-intensity exercise I experience chest tightness and sometimes I hear a wheeze. I also cough a lot afterwards. This happens all the time and I think it is just because I'm training so hard. My nose is also constantly blocked. I've tried my friend's asthma inhaler before a run and I think it might help, but I don't want to get by using inhalers. I do think if I could train and compete without my breathing symptoms I could perform better."*

Coach: *"My athlete should be able to perform better. During high-intensity efforts I can see their breathing is heavy and they need more time to recover than others. I train my athletes hard, so everyone is going to feel out of breath but this athlete is really struggling. We have tried all sorts of ways to help them complete sessions but the breathing problem is starting to impact on the overall quality and volume of the training. I may have to consider dropping them from my top training group, but this would be a real shame as they have plenty of talent."*

The above scenario is a common one in competitive sport. Our role as medical practitioners, respiratory therapists and scientists is to understand the reasons why an athlete may experience exercise-related respiratory symptoms and to ensure that a logical and robust approach is then used to diagnose, manage and monitor the issue.

The goal is to manage an athlete's problems in such a way that their respiratory health is optimised and thus any symptoms do not significantly impact on either their training or competition schedule.

Achieving this goal allows athletes to train and compete symptom-free, which will ultimately lead to improved performance and enjoyment of their chosen sport. This all seems straightforward and, in many ways obvious to state, but if this was already commonplace in medical athlete practice and we were currently perfect at optimising respiratory care of athletes, then this book would be superfluous. In our experience, the reality is that this is far from the case and respiratory problems in athletic individuals, frequently remain overlooked, poorly managed and in many cases simply dismissed.

Respiratory issues in athletes – what do we know?

We know that exercise-related respiratory symptoms are the most commonly reported medical problem in competitive athletes and that asthma or at least exercise-induced bronchoconstriction (EIB) is the most prevalent chronic disease in this group of individuals. Indeed, at a major sporting competition, it is far more likely that an athlete will underperform due to a respiratory tract infection or poorly controlled airways disease or allergies than any other issue, including issues such as acute in-competition injury.

We know that if we rely on a diagnostic approach that depends on using a symptom-based approach to assessment alone to diagnose asthma and EIB in athletes, that we will get the diagnosis wrong half of the time. i.e. you might just as well throw a coin in the air to know if the athlete with wheeze and breathlessness has asthma. Similarly, when an athlete reports acute 'infective-type' respiratory symptoms, research tells us that these symptoms are *as likely* to be arising from a multitude of conditions, including upper airway allergy or inflammation, as from bacterial infection.

We know that many athletes (and their coaches) often attribute their respiratory symptoms to de-conditioning or assume it is 'just the way you breathe' and yet it is our experience that many of these individuals will ultimately turn out to have evidence of under-treated asthma or undetected upper airway or breathing pattern problems.

We know that many respiratory issues can appear 'whimsical' or 'fleeting' and may only present or be amplified at certain times of year or on exposure to certain environments (e.g. high pollution or pollen).

Research over the past fifty years has taught us a lot about respiratory problems in athletic individuals and yet sadly most of this research has failed to translate into the provision of practical and pragmatic advice for the athlete and coach.

Improving respiratory care – a way forward

We and others have spent many years trying to promote the need for improved respiratory care for athletic individuals. Despite this, it remains a fact that athletes still often receive inconsistent support for any respiratory problems, both with respect to obtaining a correct diagnosis but also with respect to getting access to the best treatment.

We are regularly challenged by coaches and medical teams who are unable to see the value of focusing attention and time on addressing respiratory health. This is remarkable, given an apparent readiness to invest time in musculoskeletal and cardiac screening. Indeed while this is clearly important the prevalence of this type of problem is dwarfed by that of respiratory illness. Asthma/EIB is consistently found in at least 1 in 4 of the members of endurance-based sporting teams that we have worked with over the past twenty years.

Respiratory health in athletes still remains overlooked, despite the fact that 1 in 4 endurance athletes have asthma or asthma-type symptoms. Surely now it's time that we wake up to this problem and take it seriously.

It's not all bad, however; some sports teams have established comprehensive support systems, much of which is based on successfully translating the research content contained within this book. Typically, athletes involved in these settings, undergo objective screening for respiratory issues and follow-up with appropriate support to monitor the impact of any intervention and therapy. However, there are still many sports and teams that do not have well developed systems in place to screen, diagnose or monitor athlete's respiratory health. It is clear there is significant disparity in the support athletes receive regarding their airway health.

Practical and pragmatic – a book to help practitioners get it right

It is on this background that we have produced this book, with the ultimate aim of providing a practical and pragmatic guide to help clinicians, coaches, athletes and their support systems to improve respiratory care. It is hoped the contents of this book can help readers better understand the plethora of respiratory conditions experienced by athletes and help sports medicine practitioners, therapists and scientists, to develop effective practice, to best support their athletes.

We are very grateful to the world-leading practitioners and scientists who have contributed to the book. Each chapter provides a unique insight and as a collective, the authors have directly delivered respiratory care to world and Olympic champions, countless professional sporting bodies and teams, national and international anti-doping organisations and helped to shape and develop athlete support systems for world and national sports organisations. Moreover, the authors, as a group have written many of the key research papers in the past two decades, underpinning the applied practice, outlined throughout this book.

We have thoroughly enjoyed editing these contributions, to deliver an informed, one-stop guide that aims to 'translate' science from 'bench to bedside' or from 'treadmill to trackside' and acts to support athletes experiencing any type of respiratory problem. It also provides the underpinning scientific basis of respiratory anatomy and function to allow practitioners to understand the basis behind delivery of care.

We hope by reading this book you can support your athletes in achieving their goals whilst breathing more easily and breathing to win.

1

THE RESPIRATORY SYSTEM AND EXERCISE

Karl P. Sylvester

Overview

This chapter will cover:

- The anatomy and physiology of the respiratory system.
- The physiology of how we breathe and what causes breathlessness.
- How exercise influences the respiratory system.
- Simple measures that can be used to evaluate the respiratory system and detect abnormal function.
- An overview of cardiopulmonary exercise testing with focus on the respiratory response to exercise.

Introduction

The human respiratory system has evolved and adapted to ensure it serves its primary function; namely to transport the necessary oxygen required for energy generation at a cellular level and to remove waste products from this energy generation, primarily carbon dioxide. It is the latter, that is generally considered to dictate the overall functional behaviour of the respiratory system and during exercise mandates a response pattern acting to address metabolic requirements. Moreover, in highly trained athletic individuals the ability to surpass the exercise capacity of the sedentary individual places additional stress on the respiratory system and in some cases may be considered to limit exercise or impede exercise capacity (see Chapter 2). Overall however the pulmonary response patterns encountered are testament to how well the respiratory system adapts to these stresses, further demonstrating the evolutionary design of the human body to adapt to its surroundings.

The aim of this chapter is to introduce key aspects of the anatomy and physiology of the respiratory system in both untrained and trained (i.e. athletic) individuals, at rest and during exercise. The chapter also evaluates and details techniques that can be undertaken to assess the functional capability of the respiratory system to respond to the challenge of exercise.

Ventilation – how do we breathe?

Air enters the lungs via bulk flow due to a negative pressure being generated within the thoracic cage. This negative pressure is generated via contraction of the diaphragm, pulling the lungs downward and the intercostal muscles pulling the ribcage up and outward.

According to Boyle's Law, under conditions of constant temperature, there is an inverse relationship between pressure and volume. This means that if pressure decreases gas volume increases. As such, by creating a negative pressure within the chest there is an increase in gas volume. Inspiration, where gas enters the lungs, is an active process during rest and exercise. At rest, the main muscle groups involved are the diaphragm and the intercostal muscles. During exercise there is further recruitment of accessory muscles to augment respiratory function. These include the sternocleidomastoid and the scalene muscles predominantly. Other muscle groups that have been observed to be recruited during exercise include serratus anterior, pectoralis major and pectoralis minor, trapezius, latissimus dorsi, erector spinae among others.

Expiration is predominantly a passive process during rest; the diaphragm relaxes and the lungs return to a state known as the functional residual capacity (FRC) or end-expiratory lung volume (EELV). This is the state whereby the opposing elastic recoil forces of the lungs and chest wall are in equilibrium. During exercise expiration becomes a more active process, with abdominal and intercostal muscles playing a greater role.

The lungs are attached to the chest wall via the pleurae. The visceral pleurae cover each lung and the parietal pleurae attach to the chest wall. Between each pleurae is a pleural cavity which contains a thin film of serous fluid. When air enters this space the lung can partially or fully collapse and the remaining air space is termed a pneumothorax.

How is breathing controlled?

Under resting conditions, small changes in ventilatory activity is controlled by the respiratory centre within the brainstem. These structures are centred in the medulla oblongata and pons. The medulla consists of two groups of neurons known as the dorsal and ventral respiratory groups and one within the pons, the pontine respiratory group. The latter includes two areas known as the pneumotaxic centre and the apneustic centre. There are several neural inputs into the respiratory centres that react to basic concentrations of oxygen, carbon dioxide and pH, but there are other inputs such as a response to hormonal changes and the ability to consciously control ventilation via the cerebral cortex.

In terms of the control of ventilation, under normal conditions of exercise, the predominant driving factor underpinning ventilation is a direct response to an increase in circulating concentrations of carbon dioxide. A bi-product of aerobic metabolism is carbon dioxide, an increase of which is detected by the respiratory centres and there is a concomitant increase in ventilation.

As exercise intensity increases aerobic metabolism must be supplemented by anaerobic metabolism. This anaerobic metabolism produces lactic acid which must be buffered by the bicarbonate system. This buffering process produces additional carbon dioxide to that of aerobic metabolism and hence ventilation increases further. Although this has been the standard explanation for the additional carbon dioxide produced during exercise, there is some contention within the literature, a summary of which can be found in sources within the additional reading list (see below). As exercise intensity continues to increase there is a point whereby there is insufficient buffering of lactic acid and the concentration of hydrogen ions increases. At this point the increase in hydrogen ions is detected by the peripheral chemoreceptors in the carotid bodies and these now takes over control of ventilation.

WORK OF BREATHING AND THE SENSATION OF BREATHLESSNESS AND DYSPNOEA

- A sensation of breathlessness is common in both health and disease and can be caused by a number of factors.
- Dyspnoea is defined as 'a subjective experience of breathing discomfort that consists of qualitatively distinct sensations that vary in intensity'.
- It is postulated that any factor that affects either the load on the respiratory muscles, their capacity or both will increase neural drive from the medullary respiratory centre to the respiratory muscles (Figure 1.1).
- Increased neural respiratory drive is produced to ensure respiratory homeostasis.
- When respiratory load and capacity is imbalanced it results in the sensation of breathlessness (Figure 1.1).

How does airflow in the respiratory tract at rest and during exercise?

The airway tract includes the nasal cavity, larynx, large central airways (i.e. trachea and main bronchi) and smaller airways. During passive resting breathing most individuals will breathe through the nose and this pattern of ventilation is preferable; the lungs function best in warm and moist conditions and the nose, with its rich plexus of capillaries, acts to warm and humidify air from the atmosphere. The nose also acts as the first line of defence, filtering out particles and infective pathogens that have the ability to damage the lungs, via cilia and increased mucus secretion.

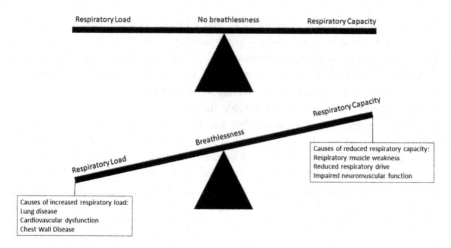

Respiratory Load   No breathlessness   Respiratory Capacity

Respiratory Capacity

Breathlessness

Respiratory Load

Causes of reduced respiratory capacity:
Respiratory muscle weakness
Reduced respiratory drive
Impaired neuromuscular function

Causes of increased respiratory load:
Lung disease
Cardiovascular dysfunction
Chest Wall Disease

FIGURE 1.1 Influence of respiratory load and capacity on breathlessness.

During exercise, as the demand to increase ventilation rises, individuals will begin (usually at approx. 35 L/min) to alter their respiratory pattern to utilise the combined oral and nasal route.

Given the resistance in the nasal cavity, it is not possible or feasible to generate sufficient airflow, via a predominant nasal breathing route, during moderate to strenuous exercise. It is therefore not logical to promote a nasal breathing pattern in athletes engaging in strenuous exercise. Moreover, there is no robust evidence that use of nasal strips or other devices to dilate the nares, is beneficial in enhancing nasal ventilation.

Any nasal obstruction arising from clinical conditions such as nasal polyps or rhinitis (see chapter 8), may force an affected individual to utilise an oral predominant breathing pattern at rest and this has deleterious implications for airway hydration, upper airway discomfort and risk of infection. As atmospheric air travels through the oro-nasal cavity there is exposure to lymphoid tissue in the form of adenoid, tubal, palatine and lingual tonsils that act as another line of defence, detecting pathogens and eliciting an immune response.

How does the larynx act as the bottleneck of the airway?

The laryngeal inlet represents a 'bottleneck' to airflow and is the last structure where there is common passage of both food and air; the lungs being protected from aspiration via the glottis. The larynx contains the vocal cords, which in conjunction with arytenoid cartilage, are used to produce sound for speech. During normal function these structures do not impact ventilation during exercise. However, in some individuals these structures may function abnormally to restrict the flow of air in and out of the lungs during strenuous exercise. Exercise-induced laryngeal obstruction (EILO) is now recognised to be highly prevalent in adolescent athletes with some studies indicating up to one in ten young athletes may have this condition, causing breathing difficulties during exercise (see Chapter 9).

What path does the air take to move from the trachea into the lungs?

Air enters the more distal airway tract via the trachea, which is a cartilage rich structure containing cilia and rich in seromucus glands, acting as another line of defence aiming to prevent pathogens and particles from entering the lungs. The trachea then divides into the two primary bronchi and this continued bifurcation continues all the way down to the alveolar ducts where the majority of gas exchange takes place. Weibel's model of the airways classifies each bifurcation of the airways as one generation. There are approximately 23 generations of the airways with air travelling via bulk flow through the conducting airways down to approximately generation 16–17. From here air travels to the alveoli via diffusion and from this point onwards gas exchange begins to take place with the major gas exchange occurring within the alveolar ducts and individual alveoli.

With increasing airway generation there is a reduction in cartilage tissue. Airway tone is thus maintained via an increase in smooth muscle, which under normal conditions contracts and relaxes appropriately to external factors. In the presence of heightened bronchial hyper-responsiveness, there is an exaggerated smooth muscle response with increased smooth muscle contraction causing a reduction in airway patency that then impacts on exercise ability.

Increased exercise intensity, with a potential concomitant reduction in humidification and warming of air entering the lungs as explained above, can increase the osmolality of the airways eliciting a cascade response leading to airway constriction via exaggerated smooth muscle contraction, resulting in exercise induced bronchoconstriction. Cold air can accentuate this response. The impact and assessment is explained in further detail in later chapters (Chapters 4 and 5).

How does gas exchange take place in the lung?

Once air reaches the gas exchange zones, oxygen must diffuse across the airway epithelium into the pulmonary capillaries and combine with haemoglobin in the erythrocytes to be transported around the body. The combination of oxygen with haemoglobin takes approximately 0.25 seconds. Under resting conditions pulmonary capillary transit time is approximately 0.75 seconds and so there is sufficient time for uptake of oxygen onto the haemoglobin molecule before blood leaves the lungs. At peak exercise pulmonary capillary transit time reduces to 0.25 seconds. Therefore, again, the human body has optimally evolved to cope with increases in exercise intensity as combination of oxygen to haemoglobin and pulmonary capillary transit time are optimally matched. Where there are conditions of reduced ventilation and therefore a reduction in delivery of oxygen to the gas exchange areas of the lung, or a reduction in the ability for gases to diffuse across the alveo-lar-capillary membrane, or where there is a reduction in pulmonary capillary tran-sit/volume, there will be a reduction in oxygen delivery to exercising muscles. This will then impact on the ability of the individual to exercise to their maximum capacity through reduced oxygen delivery to exercising muscles.

AT WHAT AGE DO OUR LUNGS REACH THEIR MAXIMUM CAPACITY?

There is a rapid increase in lung capacity in early age, reaching its peak at approximately 20–25 years of age before beginning to decline (see Figure 1.2).

What tools are available to monitor and assess lung function?

We have the ability to physiologically assess whether abnormalities are present at all of the pathways outlined above using various techniques. The most commonly utilised assessment of lung function is spirometry (Association for Respiratory Technology & Physiology 2017).

This measurement can be performed as a relaxed manoeuvre giving an indica-tion of lung volume in the form of vital capacity (VC). On its own this has some utility in defining whether there is any pathology in the form of a restrictive lung disease such as interstitial lung disease (ILD). Performing the manoeuvre in both the sitting (Figure 1.3) and laying positions also gives some insight into whether there is an abnormality of respiratory muscle strength. The disadvantage to the

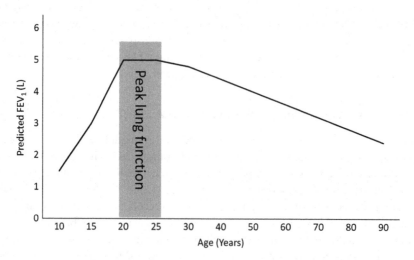

FIGURE 1.2 Changes in forced expiratory volume in one second throughout the life span of a male.

latter being a significant difference in positional spirometry only being demonstrated when there is moderate to severe muscle weakness and so early onset muscle weakness could be missed using this technique only.

Performing the same manoeuvre but using a forced technique then allows the measurement Forced Vital Capacity (FVC) and additional parameters such as the forced expiratory volume in one second (FEV$_1$; Figure 1.4). This value in combination with the ratio of FEV$_1$ to FVC or expressed as a percentage (FEV$_1$/FVC or FEV$_1$/FVC %) allows further investigation of any obstructive lung pathology such as asthma or chronic obstructive pulmonary disease (COPD). Utilising flow measuring devices further expands the parameters that can be measured to include the peak expiratory flow (PEF) or mid-expiratory flow rates (MEF$_{25-75}$, MEF$_{50}$) which enhances the ability to measure obstructive abnormalities of the smaller/peripheral airways that volumes alone occasionally do not detect. Spirometry techniques are also utilised in the context of exercise when assessing for the presence of exercise-induced abnormalities, such as exercise induced bronchoconstriction (EIB) (see Chapter 5 for further information).

To ensure accurate measurement, it is important that standardised quality assured best practice guidance is followed (see www.ARTP.com), that includes

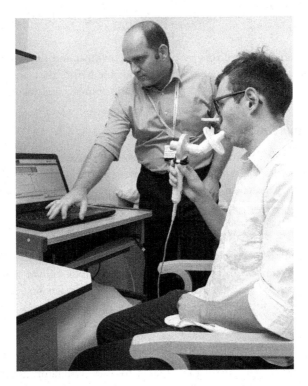

FIGURE 1.3 A patient performing spirometry.

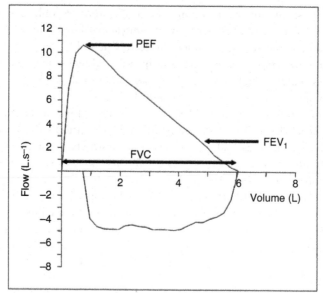

FVC = Forced Vital Capacity;
FEV_1 = Forced Expiratory Volume in One Second;
PEF = Peak Expiratory Flow

FIGURE 1.4 Forced flow-volume loop in a normal healthy participant.

detection of performance errors by both the individual and the equipment. The measurements must be acceptable and reproducible before they are accepted as a true record. Details of the quality assurance of spirometry are detailed elsewhere.

Bronchoprovocation testing

In some individuals baseline lung function assessment may produce normal results but they still experience symptoms on exercise which can influence their exercise performance. One potential cause is increased hyper-responsiveness. These would include those susceptible individuals described previously who have reduced efficiency of airway re-warming and humidification at high ventilatory rates. It is possible to assess the presence of such hyper-responsiveness through bronchoprovocation testing using stimuli such as exercise, a forced increase in ventilatory rate (eucapnic voluntary hyperventilation), inhalation of a sugar alcohol known as Mannitol or direct stimuli such as inhalation of increasing doses of methacholine. Such provocation testing will be discussed in greater detail later in the book (see Chapter 5).

How can we assess respiratory muscle function?

As explained above, spirometry can be used to assess respiratory muscle function but its utilisation is limited in mild to moderate respiratory muscle abnormalities.

Other assessment approaches are available and can be invasive or non-invasive, volitional or non-volitional.

The simplest assessment is the Sniff Nasal Inspiratory Pressure (SNIP), which requires the subject to place a small bung/nasal olive into one nostril, leave the contralateral nostril free and perform a short sharp sniff. There are limits of normality that allow determination of the presence or absence of inspiratory muscle weakness.

Other volitional non-invasive assessments of respiratory muscle strength are the maximal inspiratory (MIP) and expiratory (MEP) pressure measurements. Subjects are requested to attempt to inspire or expire maximally against a closed shutter for at least two seconds to generate the maximum pressure possible. The MEP allows determination of abnormalities on expiratory respiratory muscle strength that the SNIP does not.

All of these assessments allow the determination of global respiratory muscle strength that is the diaphragm plus all the accessory muscles to respiration. To measure diaphragm strength in isolation requires invasive procedures such as the twitch diaphragm pressure (TwPdi). This and similar measurements require balloons or pressure catheters to be passed into the oesophagus. Pressure measurements should be made within the oesophagus but also in the stomach, therefore straddling the diaphragm, the difference in these pressures giving an indication of diaphragm strength. Manoeuvres can be performed which are either volitional (i.e. a sniff) or non-volitional. Non-volitional measurements require stimulation of the phrenic nerve to cause contraction of the diaphragm. Phrenic nerve stimulation can be achieved through electrical stimulation but there can be pain associated and so more commonly stimulation is via magnetic stimulation using magnetic coils placed on top of the skin and over the phrenic nerve.

What other measurements can be helpful to understand respiratory health?

Other measures of pulmonary function include assessment of airway inflammation by assessing the fraction of exhaled nitric oxide, airway resistance, assessments of nasal flow and dynamic exercise tests evaluating laryngeal movement continuously during exercise (see Chapters 5 and 9).

How can we assess the effectiveness of the cardio-pulmonary system during exercise?

All of the assessments described above measure a particular aspect of the respiratory system in isolation and atypically at rest and thus do not evaluate the physiological response to exercise, as a whole. Physiological responses to exercise are multi-system and multi-factorial. Exercise capacity can be impaired because of defects in ventilation and gas exchange, but also in the delivery of oxygen to exercising muscles by the cardiovascular system and the oxygen extraction at the muscles. The only assessment available that has the ability to interrogate the response to exercise along the entire physiological pathway is a cardio-pulmonary exercise test (CPET). The test can be conducted in many ways utilising many exercise protocols.

The predominant ergometers of choice are the treadmill (Figure 1.5) or cycle ergometer, however, in the field of sports science exercise specific stressors are likely more relevant, e.g. rowing ergometer or even assessing the response in a pool specifically designed to assess the exercise response in swimmers (see later chapters). Any system must be able to deliver a range of set workloads to the subject performing the exercise test.

What is an effective CPET protocol?

The test can be conducted utilising a number of different protocols. An incremental ramp exercise test is the most widely utilised approach and introduces an increasing workload to the subject, starting at zero or more often with a small workload, with the load increasing in small to large increments over a period of time, e.g. a change in a set number of Watts over seconds or minutes, up to the point of subject exhaustion. The incremental protocol set will depend on the desired outcome and interim analysis required, e.g. non-invasive determination of metabolic threshold or maximal oxygen consumption (VO_{2max}).

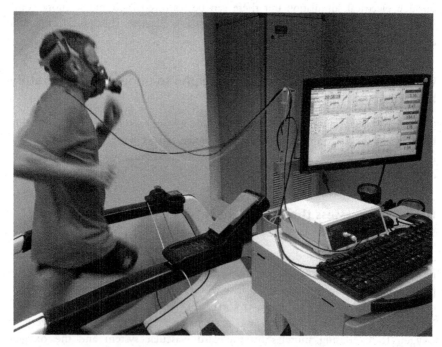

FIGURE 1.5 Athlete undergoing a cardiopulmonary exercise test (CPET) on a treadmill.

Steady state protocols require the subject to exercise at a set workload. This workload is usually selected from the maximum workload achieved during an incremental test and can be anywhere between 60–90% of the maximum achieved. The aim being to set the workload above the critical power, which is the work rate below which exercise can be sustained theoretically without fatigue with continuous energy supplementation. Steady state protocols are more appropriate than incremental tests at determining the physiological response to interventions, be these pharmaceutical or exercise training etc.

What variables can be measured during a CPET?

The main response variables measured during a CPET are the consumption of oxygen (VO_2) and carbon dioxide production (VCO_2). The cardiovascular response to exercise is measured via a 12-lead ECG and measurement of blood pressure can be included. Ventilation and the ventilatory response to exercise are also measured directly. These measured variables can be combined to create a number of calculated variables, such as oxygen pulse or ventilatory equivalents.

How do we interpret the measurement taken during the CPET?

Displaying these measured and calculated variables allows the physiological response to exercise of multiple systems to be interpreted. The most common interpretive resource for a cardio-pulmonary exercise test is the 9-panel plot. These are 9 standardised charts which display the aerobic, cardiovascular and ventilatory responses to exercise. Visual interpretation of the presence of any abnormalities is then possible, be these in oxygen delivery/extraction, with the cardiovascular or respiratory systems or in gas exchange. Detailed explanation of each of the plots and how they can be interpreted can be found in the literature and resources listed in key reading below. Once a suspected abnormality has been identified, calculation of certain parameters in relation to predicted normality allows assignment of the degree of impairment and/or the level of fitness. For instance, comparison of an individuals measured peak VO_2 to fitness categorised age and sex-grouped values allows estimation of their fitness.

Slopes can be calculated from some of the response variables to identify any specific abnormalities. Examples include the relationship between oxygen uptake and load applied as a measure of work efficiency, heart rate versus oxygen consumption as a measure of cardiovascular efficiency or ventilation versus carbon dioxide production as a measure of ventilatory efficiency.

What do the terms 'respiratory compensation point' and 'ventilatory threshold' mean?

As explained previously, there is a very close relationship between minute ventilation (V_E) and VCO_2 which, during a ramp exercise test. Even with the increased production of CO_2 through anaerobic metabolism, supplementing that produced during aerobic metabolism, the V_E and VCO_2 relationship remains linear. Only when it reaches the point whereby the production of lactic acid through anaerobic metabolism becomes too great for the bicarbonate buffering system does this relationship become non-linear and an inflection point arise. This inflection is caused by an increase in V_E out of phase with the production of CO_2 and is the result of higher levels of circulating hydrogen ions being detected by the carotid bodies which now take over the control of ventilation. Not all sedentary individuals will demonstrate this inflection of the ventilatory slope due to reduced effort and certainly those with lung disease, be this an obstructive or restrictive lung disease, will not demonstrate this inflection due to an inability to drive their ventilation rates up high enough.

An increased ventilatory (V_E/VCO_2) slope can indicate the presence of increased pulmonary dead space or indeed may be altered by a reduced $PaCO_2$ value. Elevated ventilatory equivalents provide similar insight.

Is it possible to detect disordered breathing patterns from a CPET?

A number of abnormalities may act to indicate a breathing pattern disorder of 'dysfunctional breathing' response to exercise (see chapter 11). Historically, this entity was termed hyperventilation and thus the detection of a low $PaCO_2$ was the defining characteristic. Acute hyperventilation is associated with a response pattern that includes a reduction in end-tidal carbon dioxide levels ($P_{ET}CO_2$) and a raised Respiratory Exchange Ratio (RER = VCO_2/VO_2). In the more chronic state of hyperventilation, there may be buffering and acid–base re-balancing that leads to a chronically low $P_{ET}CO_2$, but an RER that is normal. It is important however to recognise that hyperventilation can occur as a secondary phenomenon (i.e. to a lung disease process causing hypoxaemia) and thus it is important to have an interpretive strategy that considers the differential diagnosis and oxygen response pattern to exercise.

More recently, it has been recognised that individuals might develop features of dysfunctional breathing in the absence of documented physiological evidence of systemic hypocarbia. In this instance it is useful to observe the pattern of the relationship between tidal volume (V_t) and/or breathing frequency (B_f) to ventilation (V_E). The normal response is for V_E to initially increase through a rise in V_t with little to no rise in B_f. As V_t begins to plateau the increase in V_E must now come from a greater increase in B_f. In most sedentary individuals the pattern stops here. However, in more motivated individuals V_E continues to increase but the pattern response is a reduction in V_t with a further increase in B_f. An abnormal breathing pattern response can produce a number of different changes to the expected response. This can be through deep long breaths, so a much bigger increase in V_t than expected with no change in B_f or rapid shallow breaths, so an abnormally early increase in B_f with little to no change in V_t. Often both these patterns appear during the same exercise test causing a chaotic breathing pattern response of rapid shallow breaths interspersed with long deep sighs. It is also valuable to observe the pattern of thoracic movement. i.e. apical versus basal predominant. This is covered in more depth in later chapters (see Chapter 11).

Conclusion

The human respiratory system has evolved to adapt to the enviromental and physiological challenges placed on it. There are biological processes in place to deal with the external environmental threat and pathogens and from the demand from increased loading on the system through increased activity and strenuous exercise. In certain circumstances these adaptations can be blunted or indeed fail under physiological stress and thus lead to respiratory symptoms and the pathologies that will be outlined in the subsequent chapters. To detect these abnormalities and to successfully differentiate normality from pathology it is necessary to have a good understanding of the investigations that are available. It is equally important to have a robust understanding of how to apply and interpret the results in both the resting and exercise state.

Multiple-choice questions

1. Which element of the breathing cycle is passive at rest?

    (A) Expiration
    (B) Inspiration
    (C) Both
    (D) Neither

2. In a healthy individual during low to moderate intensity exercise, what controls ventilation?

    (A) Oxygen
    (B) pH
    (C) Lactic acid
    (D) Carbon dioxide

3. What is the pulmonary capillary transit time during peak exercise?

    (A) 0.25 seconds
    (B) 0.75 seconds

(C)   2 seconds
(D)   10 seconds

4.   At what age do our lungs reach peak capacity?

(A)   15–20 years
(B)   20–25 years
(C)   25–30 years
(D)   30–35 years

5.   What does the value FEV_1 represent?

(A)   The forced expiratory volume expired in total
(B)   The forced expiratory volume expired in the first 100 ms
(C)   The forced expiratory volume in the first second of expiration
(D)   The forced expiratory volume expired in the last second

Online resources

Structure and function of the lung (John B. West): www.youtube.com/watch?v=9bfl3Jtfng8.
Lung function testing (ARTP): www.artp.org.uk/en/patient/lung-function-tests/index.cfm.
Spirometry (SpirXpert): https://spirxpert.ers-education.org/en/spirometry/welcome-to-spirxpert.
Association for Respiratory and Technical Physiology: www.artp.org.uk/en/patient/lung-function-tests/spirometry.cfm.

Key reading

Aliverti, A. (2016). The respiratory muscles during exercise. *Breathe*, 12, pp. 165–168.

Association for Respiratory Technology & Physiology. (2017). *Practical Handbook of Spirometry*. 3rd ed. Lichfield: ARTP.

ATS/ACCP. (2003). ATS/ACCP statement on cardiopulmonary exercise testing. *Am J Respir Crit Care Med*, 167, pp. 211–277.

Chambers, D. J. & Wisely, N. A. (2019) Cardiopulmonary exercise testing – a beginner's guide to the nine-panel plot. *BJA Education*, 19, pp. 158–164.

Cooper, C. B. & Storer, T. W. (2001). *Exercise Testing and Interpretation: A Practical Approach*. Cambridge: Cambridge University Press.

Cotes, J. E., Chinn, D. J. & Miller, M. R. (2009). *Lung Function: Physiology, Measurement and Application in Medicine*. 6th ed. Chichester: Wiley.

Johnson, R. L., Spicer, W. L., Bishop, J. M. & Forster, R. E. (1960). Pulmonary capillary blood volume, flow and diffusing capacity during exercise. *Journal of Applied Physiology*, 15 (5), pp. 893–902.

Nielsen, E. W., Hull, J. H. & Backer, V. (2013). High prevalence of exercise-induced laryngeal obstruction in athletes. *Medicine and Science in Sports and Exercise*, 45(11), pp. 2030–2035.

Polkey, M. I., Green, M. & Moxham, J. (1995). Measurement of respiratory muscle strength. *Thorax*, 50, pp. 1131–1135.

Rotman, H. H., Liss, H. P. & Weg, J. G. (1975). Diagnosis of upper airway obstruction by pulmonary function testing. *Chest*, 68, pp. 796–799.

Wasserman, K., Hansen, J., Sietsema, K., Sue, D., Stringer, W., Sun, X. & Whipp, B. (2011). *Principles of Exercise Testing and Interpretation: Including Pathophysiology and Clinical Applications*. 5th ed. Philadelphia, PA: Lippincott Williams & Wilkins.

Whipp, B. J. & Ward, S. A. (2011). The physiological basis of the 'anaerobic threshold' and implications for clinical cardiopulmonary exercise testing. *Anaesthesia*, 66(2), pp. 1048–1049.

Answers: 1 (A), 2 (D), 3 (A), 4 (B), 5 (C)

2

RESPIRATORY LIMITATIONS TO EXERCISE

Joseph F. Welch, Bruno Archiza and A. William Sheel

Overview

This chapter will cover:

- Introduce the concept of respiratory limitation and discuss the importance of understanding differences between demand and/or capacity issues.
- Describe the normal adaptations that occur in response to athletic training.
- Introduce the concept that airflow limitation may impact athletic performance.
- Explain how exercise-induced arterial hypoxaemia may occur and its impact on exercise performance.
- Discuss how respiratory muscle function may contribute to respiratory limitation.

Introduction

Traditionally, the respiratory system in healthy individuals has been described as 'overbuilt' for the demands placed on it during intense muscular exercise. As discussed in Chapter 1, during exercise the arterial partial pressure of oxygen (PaO_2) and carbon dioxide ($PaCO_2$) remain near to resting levels. This is due principally to the precise matching of alveolar ventilation to metabolic rate.

The structure of the lungs (e.g. large surface area and thin blood-gas barrier to maximise diffusion of gases), airways (e.g. richly innervated by β_2 adrenergic receptors to improve laminar airflow) and respiratory muscles (e.g. high oxidative capacity to prevent fatigue) are well suited to their function – a concept known as symmorphosis. However, no bodily system is without limitation. A respiratory-related threat to arterial O_2 content (C_aO_2) and convective O_2 transport may exist under certain conditions of exercise in both healthy athletic humans and in those with respiratory disease. As will be described in the later chapters in this book, both upper and lower airway disorders such as exercise-induced laryngeal obstruction (EILO), asthma and exercise-induced bronchoconstriction (EIB) respectively, may impair respiratory function and lead to exercise limitation. This chapter will examine and summarise how several conditions may impact the respiratory system and lead to exercise intolerance.

What is ventilatory limitation?

Ventilatory limitation can be defined as the presence of a state in which factors actually prevent a particular function from increasing in the face of an increased requirement for ventilation. Ventilatory constraint, on the other hand, is defined as the influence of some mechanism that opposes the requirement for ventilation and therefore induces a reduction in the achieved response but that does not, in itself, limit the system further response.

What is the concept of respiratory demand and capacity?

The demand vs. capacity theory holds that there are circumstances whereby the substantial physiological requirement mandated by vigorous exercise can meet or exceed the capacity of the respiratory system to respond. Specifically, with training, the cardiovascular and musculoskeletal systems demonstrate progressive structural and functional adaptations and yet in comparison the lungs, airways and respiratory muscles, do not exhibit this pattern of adaption to any significant degree (Table 2.1). Thus, the once considered 'overbuilt' lungs then can become a so-called 'limiting factor', affecting O_2 transport and utilisation in highly trained endurance athletes. The mismatching of physiological systems is central to the demand vs. capacity theory (i.e. as demand is increased the capacity of the respiratory system to respond is reached).

The peak capacity of the lungs to ventilatory capacity is dependent on a number of factors, including: genetic endowment, ageing and disease (e.g. EIB). On the other hand, ventilatory demand is determined by metabolic requirement, body weight and dead space ventilation.

Exercise capacity is often defined by peak oxygen uptake (O_2), defined by the Fick equation, as the product of cardiac output (CO) and the arterio-venous oxygen (CaO_2-CvO_2) difference (i.e. how much oxygen is extracted at the muscular/peripheral level). Hence, any step along the O_2 transport cascade, from the atmosphere to the mitochondria, can contribute to impaired O_2. As briefly described above, in very few instances does the healthy human pulmonary system limit C_aO_2. Obstructive airway disorders, such as asthma and EILO, however can lead to airflow limitation causing an increase in respiratory muscle work, impaired gas exchange and a perception of dyspnoea exchange impairment, all of which may reduce and compromise exercise tolerance.

TABLE 2.1 Cardio-respiratory adaptations to endurance training

System	Physiological measure	Exercise adaptation
Cardiac	Cardiac output	↑
	SV max	↑
	Heart rate max	None (↓)
	Aerobic capacity (VO2max)	↑
	Resting heart rate	↓
Blood	Hb	↑
	Plasma volume	↑
Muscle	Mitochondrial density	↑
	Oxidative enzyme activity	↑
	Capillary density	↑
Respiratory	FVC	None
	FEV_1	None
	PEF	None
	Tidal volume	None
	BF	↑
	Minute ventilation	↑
	Ventilatory efficiency	↑

What are the respiratory factors that might limit exercise tolerance in an athlete?

In the endurance-trained athlete, the pulmonary system may contribute to exercise impairment for one of four main reasons: (1) airflow limitation, (2) dyspnoea, (3) exercise-induced arterial hypoxaemia (EIAH), and (4) respiratory muscle fatigue (RMF), shown in Figure 2.1.

What is airflow limitation?

Airflow limitation is most often defined by the presence of characteristic changes on pulmonary function tests (e.g. a reduced FEV1/FVC ratio below 0.7). An alternative definition is of an abnormal decrease in the maximal expiratory flow rate at a given lung volume and thus an imbalance between demand and capacity.

Ventilatory mechanics and airflow are typically assessed via flow-volume loops (FVL) (see Chapter 1). Plotting the exercise tidal FVL within the maximal expiratory flow-volume curve (MEFV) enables respiratory physiologists to determine

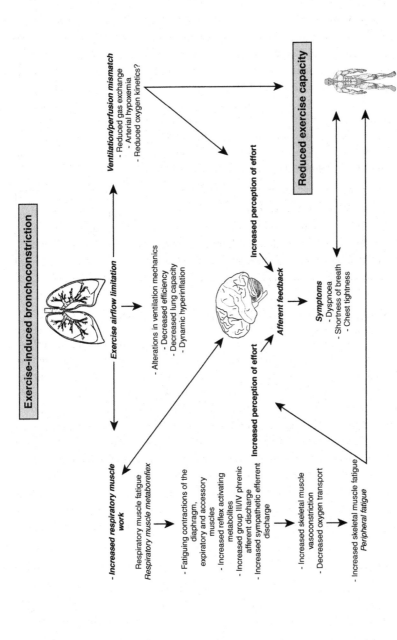

FIGURE 2.1 Proposed mechanisms of reduced exercise capacity in EIB.
Source: from Price et al. (2014)

how much ventilatory reserve remains for increased flow. Expiratory flow limitation (EFL) may be defined as failure to increase expiratory flow (Figure 2.2) despite an increase in driving pressure and can be assessed by the encroachment of the tidal FVL upon the MEFV.

In a healthy individual, during incremental exercise, end-expiratory lung volume (EELV) decreases while end-inspiratory lung volume increases. This shift in operational lung volumes minimises the mechanical work of breathing (WOB) by optimising diaphragmatic length. In the presence of EFL, however, a relative hyperinflation of the lungs occurs, thereby placing the respiratory muscles at a functional disadvantage. Diaphragm sarcomeres are shorter in length and must operate on a weaker segment of their length-tension and force-velocity relationships. As a result, force generation requires substantially more effort and can contribute to the development of RMF and dyspnoea. What's more, respiratory system compliance is reduced at high lung volumes leading to an enhanced elastic WOB.

> The work of breathing (WOB) is a major determinant of respiratory muscle fatigue, which can be influenced by mechanical ventilatory constraints, such as EFL. By breathing at higher lung volumes (as observed in asthma), neural respiratory drive is increased and subsequently WOB.

Can airflow limitation in asthma limit exercise performance?

There remains considerable debate as to whether EIB can limit exercise performance. Intuitively, the development of airway narrowing would be expected to increase WOB and hence impact total energy expenditure. However, as will be covered in subsequent chapters, asthma and EIB are typically associated with reductions in airway calibre in the post exercise phase. Indeed studies have shown that the pre-exercise development of bronchoconstriction (e.g. by getting an asthmatic to undertake a bronchoprovocation challenge before then exercising) are not typically associated with large impairments in pulmonary function. This acknowledged, the development of EIB can lead to compromised alveolar ventilation and exchange of O_2 and CO_2 at the blood gas barrier. It can also lead to the development of dyspnoea and this may impact an athlete's ability to exercise (Figure 2.2). Similar findings may be relevant in EILO, covered in Chapter 9.

What is dyspnoea?

Dyspnoea is defined as subjective experience of breathing discomfort that consists of qualitatively distinct sensations that vary in intensity. Multifaceted and highly complex, dyspnoea derives from interactions among multiple physiological, psychological, social, and environmental factors that may induce secondary physiological and behavioural responses. During exercise, this 'shortness of breath' worsens as exercise intensity increases, requiring a larger WOB. Afferent mechanoreceptors signal increased central respiratory drive while effort and work sensations are also increased.

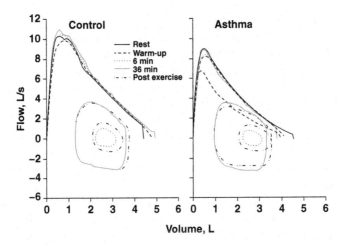

FIGURE 2.2 Flow-volume loops in healthy controls and asthmatics during constant load submaximal exercise.

Source: Johnson et al. (1995)

Dyspnoea is not considered the primary reason for exercise cessation in healthy individuals; however, as outlined above, it may play a role in impairment of performance in athletes with EIB.

What is exercise-induced arterial hypoxaemia?

Maintaining C_aO_2 during exercise is an important determinant of O_2 transport and maximal O_2. Even during maximal exercise, C_aO_2 is maintained within narrow limits because the lung and chest wall are generally 'overbuilt' with respect to the metabolic demands for gas transport. Moreover, the alveolar-arterial PO_2 difference (AaDO$_2$) widens only minimally above resting levels, meaning that O_2 diffusion across the alveolar-capillary membrane is not compromised. It is also generally observed that during strenuous exercise alveolar hyperventilation raises alveolar PO_2 in order to compensate for the widened AaDO$_2$ and as such, arterial PO_2 and oxyhaemoglobin saturation (S_aO_2) are maintained near resting levels. While the above is the general 'rule', there are notable exceptions where arterial blood gas homeostasis is not always maintained in otherwise healthy humans during exercise. Arterial O_2 desaturation of 3–15% below resting levels have been observed to occur at or near maximum exercise intensities. Most studies have reported EIAH in fit young males, as sedentary males do not experience EIAH. There are reports that women may be more susceptible to EIAH. However, this is not a universal finding and the true 'incidence' of EIAH in men or women has not been definitively established.

While EIAH typically occurs during strenuous exercise, it is underappreciated that many of those experiencing EIAH begin to show clear decrements of arterial PO_2 (because of a widened AaDO$_2$ and underventilation) even in steady-state submaximal exercise. The EIAH that occurs with submaximal exercise is most often associated with a transient hypoventilation with accompanying hypoxaemia in moderate intensity exercise, which is subsequently corrected during heavy and maximal exercise as hyperventilation occurs and the AaDO$_2$ is not abnormally widened. In athletes, EIAH during submaximal exercise is accompanied by both relative hypoventilation and a widened AaDO$_2$. These abnormalities worsen with further increases in exercise intensity, thereby reducing arterial PO_2 and S$_a$O$_2$ further.

A lowering of arterial PO_2 below rest (100 mmHg) is due to a widened AaDO$_2$ and/or insufficient increase in alveolar PO_2. Oxyhaemoglobin desaturation is further exaggerated by a rightward shift of the O$_2$ dissociation curve due to metabolic acidosis and increased temperature. The precise causes of the fall in arterial PO_2 or S$_a$O$_2$ are unclear. However, based on the available data in humans the mechanistic basis of EIAH relate to relative alveolar hypoventilation, ventilation-perfusion inequality and diffusion limitation. There are reports that exercise-induced intrapulmonary shunting may contribute to EIAH, but this is controversial and remains unresolved.

By adding increased oxygen to the inspirate, peak O$_2$ may increase 2% for every 1% reduction in S$_a$O$_2$. Preventing EIAH sufficiently to raise PO$_2$, S$_a$O$_2$ and C$_a$O$_2$ back to the normoxic range improves indices of endurance exercise performance.

One study by the authors measured arterial blood-gases and airway inflammation in mild-moderate asthmatics during treadmill exercise to exhaustion. Evidence of EIAH (SaO$_2$ ≤ 94%) was found in 38% of subjects. A widened AaDO$_2$ (i.e. gas exchange impairment) and elevated arterial PCO_2 (i.e. relative alveolar hypoventilation) accounted for the hypoxaemia. In addition, EFL was present in 90% of subjects and contributed to the inadequate ventilatory response. Exercise arterial PO_2 was lower and AaDO$_2$ wider in subjects with increased sputum histamine.

How do respiratory muscles work and can they be become fatigued?

The ability of the respiratory system to maintain blood-gas homeostasis during intense muscular exercise is challenged in the following ways:

1. oxygenation of mixed venous blood delivered to the lungs is greatly reduced;
2. pulmonary capillary red-cell transmit time decreases substantially, thereby reducing diffusion time of gases;
3. receipt of entire CO means pulmonary vascular must be controlled; and
4. a 20-fold increase in minute ventilation to match metabolic demand.

Exercise hyperpnoea is the respiratory system's first line of defence to meet these challenges, but imposes substantial requirement upon the muscles of respiration.

In order to minimise respiratory muscle work, the ventilatory response to exercise is governed by the 'principle of minimum effort'. Increased tidal volume reduces dead space ventilation at the onset of exercise, lung volumes are regulated to operate on the linear portion of the pressure-volume relationship thereby optimising compliance, accessory inspiratory muscles are recruited to relieve diaphragmatic work, and expiratory muscles assist lowering end-expiratory lung volume. However, the hyperpnoea of exercise can command between 10–15% of total O_2 depending on training status and sex, and 14–16% of maximum CO. Due to a combination of a high work of breathing, accumulation of metabolites and competition for finite CO, the respiratory muscles fatigue (RMF).

Fatigue of the muscle can be defined as a loss in the maximum force-generating capacity of a muscle during voluntary contractions whether or not the task can be sustained and is reversible by rest. The diaphragm is the principle muscle of respiration. Unlike any other skeletal muscles in the human body, the diaphragm must contract and relax continuously throughout life. A high capacity for oxidative phosphorylation and dense network of capillaries and arterial blood supply, ensures the diaphragm is well-suited for such endurance-based tasks and is therefore, highly fatigue resistant. Nonetheless, RMF does occur during short-term maximal and prolonged submaximal exercise, due to a combination of a high energetic WOB, accumulation of metabolites, and limited perfusion caused by competition for CO between respiratory and active limb locomotor muscles. Thus, the development of RMF is a function of the relationship between the magnitude of diaphragmatic work and the adequacy of its blood supply. Respiratory muscle fatigue is associated with a number of physiological consequences that may result in exercise impairment; in particular, through activation of the respiratory muscle metaboreflex (Figure 2.3).

This unique phenomenon stipulates that blood flow is preferentially redistributed away from active limb locomotor muscles in favour of the fatiguing

RESPIRATORY MUSCLE METABOREFLEX

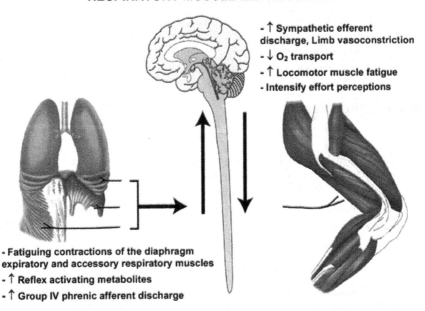

- ↑ Sympathetic efferent discharge, Limb vasoconstriction
- ↓ O_2 transport
- ↑ Locomotor muscle fatigue
- Intensify effort perceptions

- Fatiguing contractions of the diaphragm expiratory and accessory respiratory muscles
- ↑ Reflex activating metabolites
- ↑ Group IV phrenic afferent discharge

FIGURE 2.3 Respiratory muscle metaboreflex.
Source: Dempsey et al. (2006)

respiratory muscles, as has been demonstrated by unloading the respiratory muscles during exercise using proportional pressure-assist means of supporting ventilation.

Oxygen delivery to the active locomotor muscles is thusly impaired, which enhances the perception of exertion and catalyses the onset of quadriceps muscle fatigue. Through a central feedback loop, it is postulated that peripheral fatigue is confined to a 'sensory tolerance limit' via the inhibiting effects of group III/IV afferent feedback on central motor drive. Central fatigue is the result and exercise tolerance subsequently impaired.

Conclusion

The vast majority of work on respiratory system limitations to exercise have focused on the healthy human model. Disorders of the airways may contribute to exercise impairment through the effects of airflow limitation on operating lung volumes, respiratory system compliance, respiratory muscle work and subsequent cardiovascular interactions, dyspnoea, and EIAH.

Summary

- The respiratory system has historically been considered to be 'overbuilt' for purpose and thus it is often said there is 'reserve' present at the end of exhaustive exercise.
- Airway diseases such as asthma may have a significant effect on exercise capacity.
- Airflow limitation, hypoxaemia, respiratory muscle fatigue, and excessive breathlessness (or dyspnoea) are all contributory factors to the impairment of exercise performance.
- Operating lung volumes during exercise leads to augmented respiratory neural drive and a high energetic work of breathing, which may be linked with earlier onset of respiratory muscle fatigue.

Multiple choice questions

1. What are the four primary respiratory system limitations to exercise?

   (A) Airflow limitation, dyspnoea, hypoxaemia, respiratory muscle fatigue
   (B) Airflow limitation, exercise-induced bronchoconstriction, gas exchange impairment, coughing
   (C) Dyspnoea, hypoxaemia, respiratory muscle fatigue, hypoventilation
   (D) Hypoxaemia, high alveolar-arterial PO_2 difference, respiratory muscle fatigue, breathlessness

2. Dyspnoea is the subjective experience of _____?

   (A) Weakness
   (B) Hypoventilation
   (C) Breathlessness
   (D) Stridor

3. What are the potential functional consequences of airflow limitation during exercise?

   (A) Respiratory muscle fatigue, lowered work of breathing, exercise cessation
   (B) Dyspnoea, inspiratory stridor, hyperventilation, exercise intolerance, elevated work of breathing
   (C) Hypoventilation, breathlessness, hypoxaemia, inspiratory stridor
   (D) Higher operating lung volumes, elevated work of breathing, dyspnoea, respiratory muscle fatigue, exercise intolerance

4. Exercise-induced arterial hypoxaemia refers to?

   (A) A decrease in arterial O_2 saturation below resting levels
   (B) An increase in arterial O_2 saturation above resting levels
   (C) A decrease in inspired PO_2
   (D) An increase in inspired PO_2

5. Does asthma affect endurance exercise tolerance?

   (A) Yes – given the negative influence of asthma on respiration during exercise
   (B) Maybe – the mechanisms outlined in this chapter (e.g. dyspnoea, respiratory muscle fatigue) provide rationale for the potential negative influence of asthma on exercise tolerance
   (C) Maybe – the mechanisms outlined in this chapter (e.g. dyspnoea, respiratory muscle fatigue) provide rationale for the potential positive influence of asthma on exercise tolerance
   (D) No – asthma presents no influence on respiratory capacities during exercise

Key reading

Dempsey, J. A. 1986. J.B. Wolffe Memorial Lecture: Is the lung built for exercise? *Med Sci Sports Exerc*, 18, 143–155.

Dempsey, J. A., Hanson, P. G. & Henderson, K. S. 1984. Exercise-induced arterial hypoxaemia in healthy human subjects at sea level. *J Physiol*, 355, 161–175.

Dempsey, J. A., Romer, L., Rodman, J., Miller, J. & Smith, C. 2006. Consequences of exercise-induced respiratory muscle work. *Resp Physiol Neurobiol*, 151, 242–250.

Haverkamp, H. C., Dempsey, J. A., Miller, J. D., Romer, L. M., Pegelow, D. F., Rodman, J. R. & Eldridge, M. W. 2005. Gas exchange during exercise in habitually active asthmatic subjects. *J Appl Physiol*, 99, 1938–1950.

Haverkamp, H. C., Miller, J., Rodman, J., Romer, L., Pegelow, D. F., Santana, M. & Dempsey, J. A. 2003. Extrathoracic obstruction and hypoxemia occuring during exercise in a competitive female cyclist. *Chest*, 124, 1602–1605.

Jackson, A. R., Hull, J. H., Hopker, J. G. & Dickinson, J. W. 2018. Impact of detecting and treating exercise-induced bronchoconstriction in elite footballers. *ERJ Open Res*, 4, 122–2017.

Johnson, B. D., Scanlon, P. D. & Beck, K. C. 1995. Regulation of ventilatory capacity during exercise in asthmatics. *J Appl Physiol*, 79, 892–901.

Koch, S., Macinnis, M. J., Sporer, B. C., Rupert, J. L. & Koehle, M. S. 2015. Inhaled salbutamol does not affect athletic performance in asthmatic and non-asthmatic cyclists. *Br J Sports Med*, 49, 51–55.

Price, O. J., Hull, J. H., Backer, V., Hostrup, M. & Ansley, L. 2014. The impact of exercise-induced bronchoconstriction on athletic performance: a systematic review. *Sports Med*, 44, 1749–1761.

Whipp, B. J. & Pardy, R. L. 1986. Breathing during exercise. In: Macklem, P. T., Mead, J. (eds), *Handbook of physiology, section 4, vol III: Respiration*. Bethesda, MD: American Physiological Society, pp. 605–629.

Answers: 1 (A), 2 (C), 3 (D), 4 (A), 5 (B)

3

THE ENVIRONMENT AND ITS IMPACT ON RESPIRATORY HEALTH

Michael Koehle

Overview

This chapter will cover:

- The impact of the environment on the pulmonary system.
- Describe the impact of noxious airborne substances on the respiratory system; covering air pollution, altitude, cold and dry air, and the unique environment of the indoor swimming pool.
- Address the question of whether we should avoid all exercise in polluted environments.
- Review the impact of altitude and advice that should be given to athletes traveling to altitude.
- Provide strategies to avoid the deleterious effect of environment on the athletes.

Introduction

Sport and exercise takes many forms and occurs in a diverse range of environmental conditions, each providing unique stresses on the respiratory system. For example, the same individual might cycle in a climate-controlled fitness centre, on stationary bike during the winter, and then cycle to the top of an alpine climb at 2200 metres in 35-degree heat, while exposed to smoke from wildfires in the height of summer. In this example, although the form of exercise is similar, the stress placed on the respiratory system varies widely. This chapter will discuss the effects of different environments on the respiratory system and evaluate strategies to optimise exercise performance, and to minimise symptoms and adverse health consequences. We will discuss the impact of air pollution, altitude, cold and dry air, and the unique environment of the indoor swimming pool.

Where is air pollution an issue for athletes?

Air pollution can present specific challenges to athletes and really anyone undertaking exercise. Air pollution is not only a challenge confined to living in large cities, but can be present and problematic for those living in rural and remote areas. For example, smoke from wildfires, pollen, road dust and agricultural sources can be significant sources of air pollution that we do not often think of when we consider air pollution. Recent host cities for major games (e.g. the Olympic Summer Games in Beijing and Rio de Janeiro) and major sporting competitions (e.g. 2014 FIFA World Cup Final) have had sufficiently poor enough air quality to raise major concerns regarding the impact on health of the competitors and their support staff.

What makes up air pollution?

The best way to understand air pollution is to think of it as a complex mixture of gases and particles. Furthermore, pollution components can be classified as primary or secondary. A primary pollutant is a pollutant that has been emitted directly from the pollution source, such as the tailpipe of an automobile. In this example, carbon monoxide released from the car would be a primary pollutant. A secondary pollutant is created when primary pollutants are further modified in the environment after their creation. For example, ozone (O_3), is created by sunlight acting on a combination of individual pollutants. Ozone is particularly important for exercises on hot, sunny days.

The common gas components of air pollution include carbon monoxide (CO), ozone, oxides of nitrogen (NO and NO_2, referred together as NO_x) and sulphur

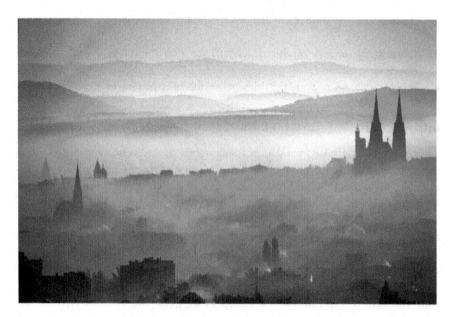

FIGURE 3.1 Visible pollution over a city.

dioxide (SO_2). Particle air pollution (termed particulate matter, or PM) is created from the combustion of fossil fuels, wood, incense, candles and certain industrial processes.

There are also natural sources of particulate matter such as wind-blown dust, pollen, and wildfires. In each situation, location, season, time of day and climate, the air pollution stimulus differs based on the sources (both indoor and outdoor) and their subsequent modification in the atmosphere. In summary, air pollution should not be considered as a single homogeneous stress, but a complicated mix of different stressors, each having individual and combined effects.

How does exercising in air pollution effect health?

Exercise places distinct challenges on the respiratory system, particularly during exposure to air pollution. As exercise intensity increases, metabolism and hence minute ventilation increases, and with it, the number of inhaled pollutants. During heavy breathing, opening the mouth becomes necessary, and the natural filtration systems of the nose and nasopharynx get bypassed. These two factors (increased ventilation and decreased filtration) lead to a dramatic increase in the dose of inhaled air pollutants, and the deposition of these pollutants in the lung, increasing the potential for adverse health effects from air pollution during exercise.

There is clear evidence that in both the long-term and short-term, air pollution has detrimental effects on health and specifically lung function. For example, PM and ozone acutely decrease tidal volume while increasing breathing frequency, and ozone also impairs lung function in healthy and asthmatic individuals. However, exercise is physiologically complex, and the combined health effects of air pollution during exercise is an area of active research.

From an overall health point of view, epidemiological studies show that exercisers in areas of higher air pollution have less health consequences than non-exercisers. Likewise, ecological studies and laboratory-controlled studies seem to find similarly that the beneficial effects of exercise are so profound, that the negative effects of air pollution can be somewhat obscured. Thus, it is clear that air pollution has clearly detrimental effects, and thus should be avoided as much as possible, with the exception of forgoing exercise. In other words, the profound beneficial effects of exercise on health seem to outweigh the negative consequences of air pollution.

SHOULD WE EXERCISE IN A POLLUTED ENVIRONMENT?

Air pollution has clearly documented harmful effects, affecting cognition, the cardiovascular system, and leading to increased risks of diseases such as cancer. Air pollution exposure should be minimised as much as possible.

However, exercise has clear beneficial health effects, and a sedentary lifestyle is a risk factor for many diseases. Instead of avoiding exercise altogether, individuals should plan their exercise in such a way to reduce pollution exposure. This involves choosing the best location and time of day to exercise when pollution dose is minimal.

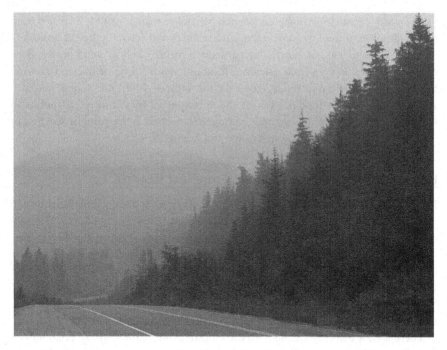

FIGURE 3.2 Cycling route on a high-pollution day, due to local forest fires.

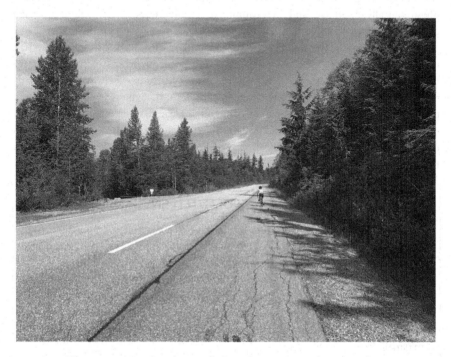

FIGURE 3.3 The same route on a low-pollution day.

How does air pollution impact on exercise performance?

From a performance point of view, there has been some observational research that has indicated a decrease in exercise performance with increased air pollution. The challenge with interpreting these types of studies is that temperature and air pollution (especially secondary pollutants such as ozone) are often correlated. Heat is well-known to affect performance, so it is not yet clear how much of the poor performance on high pollution days is due to the increase in temperature.

Does wearing a mask reduce risk of pollution exposure during exercise?

People who exercise frequently, who are often exposed to high levels of air pollution, may often choose to wear a mask, in order to reduce the pollution dose. The mask is intended to act as a filter, reducing the dose of particles retained in the lung. However, research in the area is lacking and a recent study commissioned by ANSES, the French Agency for Food, Environmental and Occupational Health & Safety, found no clear evidence of benefit for these masks, and found that instead the users had a false sense of security. For these reasons, the report recommended against the use of these masks. Clearly more research is required to assess the utility and optimal design of such a mask.

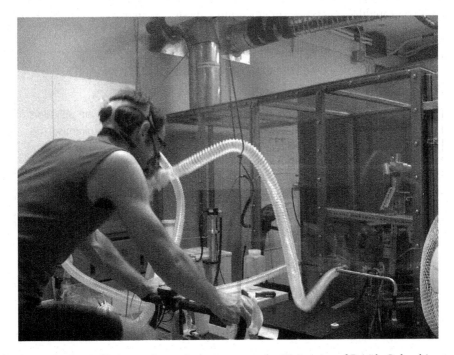

FIGURE 3.4 Air pollution and exercise exposure study, University of British Columbia. Photo: Dr Luisa Giles

Athletes often focus on outdoor air pollution only, but it is important to remember that significant air pollution exposure can occur indoors as well as outdoors. For example, in skating arenas, most ice resurfacing machines use an internal combustion engine, and can create significant levels of particulate matter, carbon monoxide and NO_2 that can affect lung function over time.

Should people with asthma exercise in air pollution?

Asthmatic athletes may be particularly concerned about the effects of air pollution during exercise, since under high pollution conditions, asthmatics are likely to be more symptomatic. Air pollution seems to dampen the natural bronchodilatory action of exercise on the lungs and increase bronchial inflammation in asthmatics. Although there is a theoretical risk that bronchodilators could enhance pollutant delivery deeper to the lung by opening up the airways, recent preliminary data indicate that salbutamol administration in asthmatics exposed to diesel exhaust does not lead to worsening of lung function when compared to placebo administration. As such, asthmatics should ensure to take their asthma medications as prescribed and in accordance with current guidelines for management of asthma. However, asthmatics should be aware that they could be more affected than their peers by air pollution, and should be extra careful to minimise air pollution exposure as much as possible during training and competition.

PRACTICAL RECOMMENDATIONS: AIR POLLUTION AND EXERCISE

1. Athletes, exercisers and event organisers should use local air pollution forecasts when planning events and training sessions to minimise the exposure to participants as much as possible.
2. Individuals should aim to exercise at times during the day when air pollution is lowest, (i.e. early in the morning, and late evening).
3. If possible, exercisers should choose locations for training and competition away from pollution sources. All individuals should remember that significant air pollution can occur both indoors and out.
4. There is some evidence that shorter, higher-intensity exercise bouts may be less detrimental than longer low-intensity sessions.
5. Individuals with pre-existing respiratory or cardiovascular disease should seek the guidance of a physician prior to starting an exercise programme, especially if there is potential for significant air pollution exposure.

How does exercising at altitude compromise exercise performance?

Athletes often train and compete at altitude, and recreational exercisers commonly seek high altitude locations for activities such as trekking, skiing and hiking. At altitude, the oxygen fraction of the air is unchanged, but the ambient barometric pressure is reduced, resulting in a lower partial pressure of inspired oxygen, and at the same time less dense, or 'thinner' inspired air. However, these stressors are often combined with cold, dry air, and potentially an austere location, which present combined challenges to the respiratory system, especially during exercise.

To ensure adequate oxygen delivery both during rest and during exercise, a variety of strategies are used by various systems of the body. Almost immediately, there are increases in both ventilation and cardiac output in order to increase the oxygen tension in the blood. Later on, there are changes in terms of chemosensitivity that allow for this increased ventilation to be maintained despite a drop in the partial pressure of carbon dioxide in the blood. This increased ventilation, especially in dry conditions can lead to an increase in insensible water losses, and the potential for dehydration.

The challenge of altitude needs to be considered in individuals with asthma, however if well managed it does not seem to pose a risk. In fact, there is no good

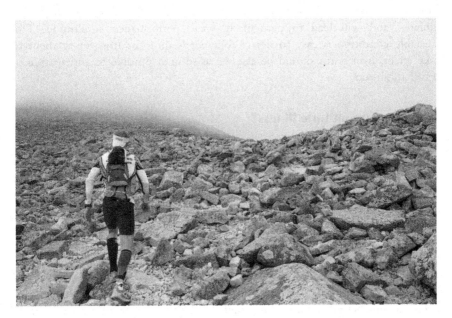

FIGURE 3.5 Athlete facing the challenges of competing at altitude; including issues from hypoxia, cold and dry air.

Photo: © Komelau | Dreamstime.com

evidence of increased symptoms or frequency of asthma attacks at altitude. Ensuring good clinical control is key before any asthmatic travels to altitude.

Historically many 'asthma rehabilitation hospitals or retreats' were deliberately placed at altitude. This phenomenon may relate to a decrease in allergen burden at altitude (i.e. the presence of house-dust mite is very low above 1500 m altitude), however, there are some cautionary points for asthmatics travelling and exercising at altitude. Firstly, visitors to altitude are often in remote, austere locations far from medical care. As such, it is advisable to bring extra medications in case of loss or inhaler malfunction. Furthermore, metered dose inhalers may not work as consistently under conditions of low temperature and low pressure. Therefore, users of inhalers are advised to keep them at all times in an inner pocket in their clothing in order to maintain a more stable temperature. Thirdly, altitude travel can often occur in parts of the world where indoor air pollution is significant from wood burning and liquefied natural gas stoves. Therefore, the asthmatic athlete may not be adversely affected by the hypoxia of altitude as much as the particulates and other pollutants to which they are exposed while indoors at altitude. Finally, other symptoms and conditions can present at altitude that may cause dyspnoea (e.g. high-altitude pulmonary oedema – HAPE) and may complicate diagnosis of an asthmatic attack or other respiratory condition.

Although not unique to those with respiratory conditions, low levels of iron stores, or even frank iron deficiency anaemia is common in endurance athletes, and will lead to particularly weak performance at altitude. This treatable condition is easy to detect, but needs time for iron replacement to take effect. Iron status should be assessed as soon as possible in anticipation of travel to altitude.

What is acute altitude illness?

All travellers and athletes at altitude are at risk of acute altitude illness (including acute mountain sickness, HAPE and high-altitude cerebral oedema – HACE). There is some evidence for a genetic predisposition for these conditions, but the most important risk factor would be rate of ascent. Fitness is not protective against altitude illness, and older individuals are not at increased risk of becoming ill.

Acute altitude illnesses can infrequently occur above 2500 metres elevation, but are much more common above 3000 metres. All three acute altitude illnesses are performance-limiting, but HAPE and HACE are much more serious and can frequently be fatal. For travel to, and events above 2500 metres, event organisers and training camp staff should have access to a clinician with a working knowledge of the diagnosis and management of these conditions. A good resource for this information is the Wilderness Medical Society Consensus Guidelines on the Prevention and Treatment of Altitude Illness. Many groups and travellers choose to bring a pulse oximeter along with them to monitor arterial oxygenation, perhaps with the goal of diagnosing altitude illness. There is much inter-individual variation in arterial oxygenation at altitude, and therefore a single measurement of oxygen saturation is quite variable in its utility for predicting and diagnosing altitude illness. However, the more serious altitude illnesses (HAPE and HACE) are associated with profound desaturation. Thus, oximetry is most useful when monitored long-itudinally in order to detect intra-individual trends in oxygenation. If one person has a sudden drop in oxygenation without a significant change in altitude, they merit special attention, and if necessary, treatment.

The best form of prevention of these acute altitude illnesses is a gradual ascent and proper acclimation to the altitude achieved before intense efforts occur. However, this approach takes time and resources, and many athletes and teams may be limited in either or both. Instead, they may seek medical advice for pro-phylactic medications to prevent altitude illness. However, the key preventive medications (such as dexamethasone and acetazolamide) are on the World Anti-Doping Agency's (WADA) Prohibited List, and thus cannot be prescribed to competitive athletes who may be governed by WADA. Therefore, prescribing practitioners need to consider the doping ramifications of these medications when counselling athletes who go to high altitude.

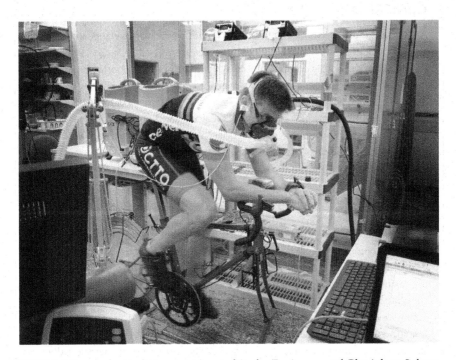

FIGURE 3.6 Research simulating exercise at altitude, Environmental Physiology Laboratory, University of British Columbia.
Photo: UBC Faculty of Medicine

PRACTICAL RECOMMENDATIONS: EXERCISE AT ALTITUDE

1.   Ensure that all individuals have received appropriate vaccinations for the high-altitude region to which they are travelling.
2.   Individuals should bring extra medication supplies, and should ensure that they keep their metered-dose inhalers in an inside pocket of their clothing, especially under cold conditions.
3.   If above 2500 metres, appropriate knowledge, medications and contingency plans are required for the prevention and management of acute altitude illness.
4.   Be aware of significant sources of pollution (indoor and outdoor) that may compromise respiratory status, training, and recovery while at altitude. Avoid these pollution sources as much as is feasible.
5.   Early detection and treatment of iron deficiency and low iron stores is essential for optimising performance at altitude.

CLINICAL CASE STUDY

A 28-year-old cyclist who lives at sea level comes to you for guidance in anticipation of competing at a multi-day cycling stage race at altitude. She lives at sea level, but has previously competed at this event and suffered poorly, noticing that her breathing had been particularly noticeable. She also had difficulty sleeping. She is otherwise well, with no history of respiratory disease and takes no medications. Her supplements include vitamin D, calcium and omega-3 fatty acids. Her diet is balanced. How would you assess her? What recommendations would you advise? (N.B. The typical medications used for the treatment and prevention of altitude illness are prohibited substances according to the WADA Code.)

Resolution

Physical examination was normal. Pulmonary function testing was normal. Eucapnic voluntary hyperpnea (EVH test) was normal. Laboratory testing ruled out iron deficiency and anaemia. The cyclist was recommended to travel to altitude approximately one week before the competition in order to partially acclimate to the altitude, overcome some of the altitude effects such as dehydration. This early arrival would help to improve her sleep, and help her to adjust to the sensations of training and competing at that altitude. She was also given a prescription for a sleeping medication that improves sleep quality and blood oxygenation during sleep, and that is permitted for use with elite sport (temazepam). The athlete followed these recommendations, and experienced a stronger performance and less symptoms than on her prior experiences at this event.

How does a cold and dry environment impact lung function?

Asthma and exercise-induced bronchoconstriction are extremely common in endurance athletes and it appears that the prevalence of bronchial hyper-responsiveness increases over the course of an endurance athlete's career. In fact, it has been recently shown that endurance athletes who require bronchodilator medications win a higher proportion of Olympic medals in endurance sports such as swimming and cycling than those who do not, despite no clear performance enhancing effects of these medications, even in athletes with EIB. Furthermore, airway hyper-responsiveness seems to occur more in winter sports athletes, and more so during the colder seasons, indicating that the cold air may play a role in the pathogenesis of this phenomenon.

The mechanisms of acute bronchoconstriction during exercise are not entirely clarified. However, it is believed that the prolonged high minute ventilations of endurance exercise can lead to respiratory heat loss, which is more pronounced when cold air is inhaled, as in winter sports. Alternatively, the high ventilation of exercise leads to enhanced water loss from the bronchial mucosa, leading to the release of mediators such as histamine and eicosanoids, causing bronchoconstriction (see Chapter 4). Cold air can carry less water vapour, and hence under cold conditions, the drying of the airways is even more pronounced. Exposure to cold air below $-20°C$ has been shown to precipitate bronchoconstriction, and as such it has been recommended that events and interval workouts not be held at temperatures colder than $-15°C$. Likewise, warming facemasks designed for sport have been created (Jonas Sport, Tenoterm) and seem to protect lung function during exercise in very cold conditions, without leading to significant excess breathing resistance.

Over time, these stresses caused by prolonged high ventilations of relatively cold and dry air on the airways can lead to the increase in prevalence of asthma that is seen in endurance athletes. It is believed to be as a result of epithelial damage that occurs during the exercise bout that accumulates over time, leading to remodelling of the airways. This phenomenon has been called 'athlete's asthma' and 'ski asthma' and appears to be potentially reversible with the cessation of endurance training.

What is the impact of swimming in chlorinated pools on lung function?

Although athletes from all endurance sports seem to be predisposed to airway hyper-responsiveness over the course of their career (as with cold weather athletes), swimmers exposed to chlorinated pools seem to be at a particularly increased. The reasons for this remain unclear but may include the prolonged endurance training at high minute ventilations involved in swimming, but additionally, the chlorine in many swimming pools may also contribute to the development of airway injury, promoting the developing of hyper-responsiveness (see Chapter 4). This notion is supported by data indicating that although the prevalence of either EIB or airway hyperresponsiveness in swimmers is similar to non-swimmers at the onset of their swimming career, the prevalence in competitive swimmers rises over the course of their athletic career.

It is important to note that EIB and airway hyperresponsiveness are not the only causes of breathing problems in swimmers. Swimmers are particularly afflicted due to the irritation caused by inhaled water droplets, and possibly the irritant effect of the chlorinated water and this may also precipitate sino-nasal problems (see Chapter 8).

Conclusion

Although the varying environments in which sport is conducted can present differing challenges to the athlete and exerciser, some practical strategies can be beneficial to minimise health consequences and optimise performance.

Summary

1. Exercisers should separate themselves from air pollution as much as possible in both time and space.
2. Proper acclimatisation is the best way to prevent the adverse health and performance effects of high altitude. This takes time.
3. Individuals with pre-existing respiratory conditions should seek medical advice in advance of exercise in a challenging environment.
4. A proper warm-up with high intensity efforts is important especially in challenging environments, and in individuals with asthma

Multiple-choice questions

1. During heavy exercise, the dose of inhaled pollution can be higher. Why?

    (A) There is more mouth breathing, allowing the inhaled pollutants to bypass filtration by the nose.
    (B) The body is moving more quickly and coming into contact with more particles.
    (C) More air is breathed in and out, leading to more pollutants getting deposited.
    (D) Both (A) and (C) are true.

2. All of the following are sources of particulate matter, except:

    (A) generation of ozone from nitrogen dioxide and hydrocarbons
    (B) wood and fossil fuel combustion
    (C) incense and candle burning
    (D) wind-blown dust and wildfires

3. Which statement is *false*:

    (A) Acetazolamide is a good choice for preventing illness and improving performance in elite athletes.
    (B) Asthmatics often have more symptoms at moderate altitude than at sea level.
    (C) Acute altitude illness typically occurs at elevations higher than 2500 metres.
    (D) Preparing for a trip to high altitude includes ensuring that all vaccinations are up-to-date.

4. Which of the following is the best predictor of the risk of acute altitude illness?

   (A) Genetic predisposition
   (B) Rate of ascent
   (C) Fitness
   (D) Age

5. Prior to exercise in the cold, asthmatics should consider all of the following, except:

   (A) Masks that help to heat and humidify the air
   (B) A structured warm-up with short intervals of high intensity exercise
   (C) Modifying the workout if extremely cold (below −15 degrees)
   (D) Ensure that the medication inhaler is at the same temperature as the environment before use

Online resources

Altitude medicine: www.altitude.org/home.php
Training in high pollution: https://youtu.be/aWTMROhJ3nk
www.csipacific.ca/2015/07/07/general-recommendations-for-athletes-training-in-bc-regions-affected-by-smoke

Key reading

Andersen, Z.J., de Nazelle, A., Mendez, M.A., Garcia-Aymerich, J., Hertel, O., Tjønneland, A., Overvad, K., Raaschou-Nielsen, O., Nieuwenhuijsen, M.J. 2015. A study of the combined effects of physical activity and air pollution on mortality in elderly urban residents: the Danish diet, cancer, and health cohort. *Environ. Health Perspect.* 123, 1–8.

Fitch, K. 2015. Air pollution, athletic health and performance and the Olympic Games. *J. Sports Med. Phys. Fitness*, 56(7–8), 922–932.

Giles, L.V., Koehle, M.S. 2014. The health effects of exercising in air pollution. *Sports Med.* 44, 223–249.

Giles, L.V., Brandenburg, J.P., Carlsten, C., Koehle, M.S. 2014. Physiological responses to diesel exhaust exposure are modified by cycling intensity. *Med. Sci. Sport. Exerc.*, 46, 1999–2006.

Grissom, C.K., Jones, B.E. 2017. Respiratory health benefits and risks of living at moderate altitude. *High Alt. Med. Biol.*, 19(2), 109–115.

Koch, S., Carlsten, C., Guenette, J.A., Koehle, M.S. 2018. Forced expiratory volume in 1 second is not affected by exposure to diesel exhaust and cycling exercise in individuals with exercise-induced bronchoconstriction. Retrieved from https://ehp.niehs.nih.gov/doi/abs/10.1289/isesisee.2018.O01.03.61

Koehle, M.S.M.S., Cheng, I., Sporer, B. 2014. Canadian Academy of Sport and Exercise Medicine position statement: athletes at high altitude. *Clin. J. Sport Med.* 24, 120–127.

Kubesch, N.J., de Nazelle, A., Westerdahl, D., Martínez, D., Carrasco-Turigas, G., Bouso, L., Guerra, S., Nieuwenhuijsen, M.J. 2015. Respiratory and inflammatory responses to short-term exposure to traffic-related air pollution with and without moderate physical activity. *Occup. Environ. Med.* 72, 284–293.

Luks, A.M., McIntosh, S.E.S.E., Grissom, C.K.C.K., Auerbach, P.S., Rodway, G.W., Schoene, R.B.R.B., Zafren, K., Hackett, P.H.P.H. 2010. Wilderness Medical Society consensus guidelines for the prevention and treatment of acute altitude illness. *Wilderness Environ. Med. J.* 21, 146–155.

MacInnis, M.J.M.J., Koehle, M.S.M.S. 2016. Evidence for and against genetic predispositions to acute and chronic altitude illnesses. *High Alt. Med. Biol.* 17(4), 284–293.

Stickland, M.K., Rowe, B.H., Spooner, C.H., Vandermeer, B., Dryden, D.M.. 2012. Effect of warm-up exercise on exercise-induced bronchoconstriction. *Medicine and Science in Sports and Exercise*, 44(3), 383–391.

Answers: 1 (D), 2 (A), 3 (B), 4 (B), 5 (D)

4

EPIDEMIOLOGY AND PATHOPHYSIOLOGY OF EXERCISE-INDUCED BRONCHOCONSTRICTION IN ATHLETES

Pascale Kippelen and Andrew Simpson

Overview

This chapter will cover:

- The key facts and figures regarding asthma and exercise-induced broncho-constriction (EIB) in athletes.
- The type of athletes who appear most susceptible to the development of EIB.
- The pathophysiology of asthma/EIB in athletes and discusses the different reasons proposed and a unified hypothesis.
- An introduction to the concept of 'airway injury' as a model to explain why athletes are more susceptible to the development of EIB.
- How to assess airway inflammation and injury.

Introduction

Asthma and exercise-induced bronchoconstriction (EIB) are frequently reported in athletes, especially in those competing at high level in endurance, winter or pool-based sports. In this chapter, we describe and address the pathophysiology and epidemiology of asthma/EIB, in various athletic populations. We then explore the mechanisms underlying EIB in athletes and consider how our current understanding of the pathophysiology of EIB informs clinical practice and may act to help us protect athletes' health.

What is exercise-induced bronchoconstriction?

Exercise-induced bronchoconstriction describes a transient narrowing of the airways that occurs in response to strenuous exercise. While often associated with asthma, EIB can occur in otherwise healthy individuals, in particular in children, members of the armed forces and athletes.

The term 'exercise-induced bronchoconstriction' is favoured over 'exercise-induced asthma', because EIB provides a physiological description of what actually occurs (i.e. narrowing of the airways) and exercise doesn't actually induce the clinical disease state of 'asthma'. Individuals with EIB typically experience respiratory symptoms, such as cough, chest tightness, breathlessness and / or mucus hypersecretion during exercise. However, these symptoms are not specific to the condition (as they can be reported by individuals without EIB, particularly during strenuous exercise).

Who gets EIB?

An increased prevalence of EIB has been repeatedly documented in a variety of athletic populations, including college, high school and recreational athletes but it is widely accepted that the prevalence of asthma / EIB is higher in elite athletes. **Indeed, it is estimated 8% of Olympic athletes suffer from asthma and/or EIB, making asthma/EIB the most common chronic medical condition in elite sport.**
Although the overall prevalence of asthma/EIB in Olympic athletes is not too dissimilar to the prevalence of asthma in the general population, the value varies widely (from <5% to ~70%) depending on the diagnostic methodology employed (i.e. symptom-based diagnosis or objective evidence of variable airflow obstruction) and the population studied. Indeed, in a study conducted in ~150 winter sports elite athletes, a symptom-based diagnosis of EIB was shown to be no more accurate than a coin toss, when compared with an objective means of diagnosis (i. e. fall in expiratory airflow, as measured by spirometry, post-exercise). Moreover, studies that have used objective means (i.e. airway reversibility to an inhaled β_2-agonist, or positive response to a direct or indirect bronchial challenge; see Chapter 5) to estimate prevalence of asthma/EIB in athletic populations show that the distribution of asthma/EIB is largely skewed across sports, with the highest prevalence observed in endurance, winter and pool-based sports. Whilst the risk for asthma/EIB development is generally lower in stop-and-go sports compared to endurance sports, in some elite football and rugby teams prevalence of 20–30% have been reported. Therefore, asthma/EIB cannot be dismissed in this category of sports.

Are endurance sports athletes more susceptible than other groups of athletes?

One of the earliest studies that showed EIB was more common in endurance-trained athletes was conducted in Scandinavian elite track and field athletes. In that study, about a quarter of long distance runners reported current asthmatic symptoms and had increased airway hyper-responsiveness or physician-diagnosed asthma compared to 4% of control individuals. Furthermore, the occurrence of asthma was

~10% higher in endurance athletes compared to speed and power athletes (incl. sprinters, throwers, jumpers and decathletes).

Subsequent data gathered from various Olympic teams and over several Olympic cycles confirmed the increased prevalence of asthma/EIB in endurance sports, with ~15–25% of endurance athletes suffering from asthma-like problems. This high rate of asthma/EIB in endurance sports is associated with a widespread use of asthma medication, in particular permitted inhaled β_2-agonists, by elite endurance athletes.

The usage of inhaled β_2-agonists is however highly variable across national Olympic teams. When, on average, 17% of Olympians from Great Britain, New Zealand and Australia declared usage of permitted inhale β_2-agonists at the 2000 and 2004 Summer Games, none of their Russian, Chinese or Korean counterparts did so. The reason for this remains unclear however may be attributable to both, variations in national prevalence of asthma (with the use of asthma medication grossly tracking prevalence rates of asthma in the general population), and national differences in respiratory health care provision (with systematic screening for asthma/EIB done in some, but not all Olympic teams) and team selection policy.

Does EIB affect winter sport athletes?

Asthma/EIB is frequently reported among elite winter sports athletes. However, as in summer sports, the distribution of asthma/EIB is not equal between athletes from various disciplines (Table 4.1) and between countries.

Among all Olympic winter disciplines, it is in cross-country skiing (i.e. the epitome of endurance sport) that the prevalence of asthma/EIB is the highest (with some reports of prevalence >50% and a large majority of skiers reporting cough on training in winter). Between 2002 and 2010, the average proportion of cross-country skiers authorised to use a permitted inhaled β_2-agonist (based on objective evidence of asthma/EIB) at the Winter Olympic Games was ~17%. Furthermore, based on medication records, the prevalence of asthma/EIB is four times higher in Olympic Nordic combined skiers who cross-country ski and ski jump (prevalence of 13%) compared with athletes who specialise in ski jumping alone (prevalence of 3%). Based on these data, the endurance element of the training is most likely responsible for the high occurrence of asthma/EIB in Nordic combined athletes.

In addition to the type of training, the cold air environment has also been shown to influence the risk of asthma/EIB occurrence in winter athletes. When the prevalence of asthma [defined as presence of asthma symptomatology, airway hyper-responsiveness (AHR) to methacholine and clinically-diagnosed asthma treated with inhaled corticosteroids] was compared between Swedish and Norwegian cross-country skiers, the value was significantly higher in Swedish (43%) compared with Norwegian athletes (14%); an observation attributed to the divergent climates (with the colder and drier climate of inland Sweden believed to increase the risk for so-called 'ski asthma').

TABLE 4.1 Examples of sports with high, medium and low risk of exercise-induced bronchoconstriction

	Risk of exercise-induced bronchoconstriction				
	High			Medium	Low
Sport category	Endurance	Winter	Pool-based	Stop-and-go	Strength and power
Examples of disciplines	Running Cycling Triathlon	Cross-country skiing Biathlon Nordic combined Speed skating Ice hockey	Swimming Synchronised swimming	Soccer Rugby	Sprinting Throwing Jumping (incl. ski jumping) Weight lifting Gymnastics Boxing Luge
Common asthma phenotype	'Atopic asthma'	'Ski asthma' or 'sports asthma'	'Sports asthma'	'Atopic asthma'	N/A

In ice-rinks sports, a 20–50% prevalence of asthma/EIB has been reported. An accelerated decay in resting lung function was also noted in young female ice-hockey players. Since concentrations of fine and ultrafine particulate matter (PM_1) in indoor ice arenas using fossil-fuelled ice resurfacing machines can be as much as twenty times greater than outside air (or in ice-rinks resurfaced with electrical-powered machines), the combined effects of endurance training and inhalation of cold, polluted air is likely to contribute to the development of respiratory dysfunction in ice-rink athletes.

Are swimmers more susceptible to EIB?

The warm and humid environment encountered by swimmers is in stark contrast to the cold dry environment typically experienced by winter athletes. Thus, historically, many young asthmatic individuals were encouraged to partake in swimming as a sporting activity of preference. Yet, it is well established that a large proportion (up to 70%) of elite swimmers are hyper-responsive to methacholine, and that pool-based athletes frequently experience exercise-induced respiratory symptoms. Indeed, pool-based and winter athletes are three and nine times, respectively, more at risk of 'sports asthma' (i.e. presence of positive asthma symptomatology and AHR) compared with other athletes. Furthermore, four of the five sports with the largest proportion of athletes seeking permission to use asthma medication at the Summer Olympic Games in 2004 and 2008 contained a swimming element (with 25% of triathletes, 17% of swimmers and modern pentathletes, and 13% of synchronised swimmers authorised to use inhaled β_2-agonists at those Games). In swimmers, it appears likely that the combination of endurance training with chronic exposure to chlorination by-products drive the development of airway dysfunction (see Chapter 3).

Does EIB develop during the course of an athletic career?

Young athletes generally appear less at risk of asthma or EIB than adult athletes. Unlike the general population who tend to display asthma in childhood and in whom EIB in childhood is often a precursor of asthma in early adulthood, the onset of EIB appears later in the life of elite athletes. Indeed, more than a third of athletes with asthma/EIB competing at the 2008 Summer Olympic Games first noted asthma symptoms after the age of 25. Similarly, half of athletes with asthma/ EIB competing at the 2006 Winter Olympic Games reported the first occurrence of respiratory symptoms on exertion after 20 years of age. Nonetheless, in some sports such as swimming, increased prevalence of asthma/EIB (>30%) have been reported in youth athletes.

Pathophysiology of EIB in athletes

Why do athletes develop EIB?

The increased prevalence of EIB in elite endurance sports is commonly attributed to the high minute ventilation (up to 200 L.min$_{-1}$) that athletes reach and sustain while exercising. High ventilatory requirements during exercise are met by an increase in breathing rate and tidal volume, as well as a shift from nasal to mouth breathing (see Chapter 1). While facilitating ventilation, mouth breathing bypasses the humidifying and heating system of the nose. Consequently, the conditioning of large volumes of air occurs further down the respiratory tract. This postponed conditioning of the inspired air leads to two major events: the cooling and the dehydration of the intra-thoracic airways. Both these events have been proposed – in the thermal and osmotic theory of EIB, respectively – to be responsible for airway narrowing.

The thermal theory of EIB

According to the thermal theory of EIB, proposed by McFadden, the cooling of the airways during exercise is followed by a rapid rewarming when exercise ceases and ventilation drops. The rapid rewarming is then thought to initiate a reactive (or rebound) hyperaemic vascular response, with capillary leakage and oedema of the airway wall, resulting in a thickening of the mucosa and narrowing of the airways.

As athletes are not able to condition air more effectively than non-athletes, yet sustain higher ventilation rates during exercise, exaggerated thermal losses and reactive hyperaemia are likely to occur, thereby increasing the risk for EIB. Further, as airway cooling is exaggerated in cold weather, winter athletes are more likely to develop EIB. However, EIB has been demonstrated to occur when hot dry air is inhaled; therefore, thermal changes alone cannot explain EIB.

The osmotic theory of EIB

According to the osmotic theory of EIB, proposed by Anderson and colleagues, it is the loss of water (not of heat) by evaporation from the airway surface during the conditioning of large volumes of inspired air over a short period of time that primarily triggers EIB. The loss of water within the intra-thoracic airways is thought to create a hyper-osmotic environment that initiates the release of bronchoconstrictive agents.

Inspired air is conditioned in the respiratory tract so that it reaches 37°C and 100% humidity by the time it reaches the alveoli. The greater the ventilation, the greater the demand on the airways to provide moisture to condition inspired air. Consequently, during heavy exercise, moisture loss from the airways extends distally, resulting in dehydration of the small airways and causing a transient increase in airway surface liquid (ASL) osmolarity. Many cells within the distal airways (including mast cells, eosinophils, epithelial cells, glandular cells and sensory nerves) are sensitive to changes in ASL osmolarity. During strenuous exercise, activation of these cells leads to the release of a wide range of inflammatory mediators – including histamine, Prostaglandin D2 (PGD_2) and cysteinyl leukotrienes (cysLTs) – which then may cause the airway smooth muscle to contract and the airways to narrow. In support to this theory, increased concentrations of histamine, PGD_2 and cystLTs have repeatedly been measured in plasma, induced sputum and urine following bronchial challenges with exercise or its surrogate (i.e. hyperpnoea of dry air) in patients with asthma and athletes with EIB.

The unifying theory of EIB

The unifying theory of EIB brings together the thermal and osmotic theories and, by doing so, helps to better understand why winter endurance athletes are at increased risk for EIB. Cold air is always dry. Hence, cold air breathing during exercise can increase the severity of EIB *via* two pathways; first, by increasing the thermal gradient post-exercise (thereby amplifying the vascular response); and second, by potentiating the dehydration of the airways – ensuing in a stronger osmotic stimulus and stronger inflammatory response (Figure 4.1).

Airway injury

Alongside thermal and osmotic changes, airway epithelial injury is thought to contribute to the development of EIB and AHR in elite athletes.

As elite (endurance) athletes reach high ventilatory rates when exercising, the smaller airways are recruited into the conditioning process. Dehydration-injury of the airway epithelium could therefore occur at the level of the small airways, triggering a complex repair process that leads, among others, to release of bulk plasma. In athletes who train daily, chronic exposure of the airway smooth muscle to the many biologically active agents present in the plasma (such as cytokines,

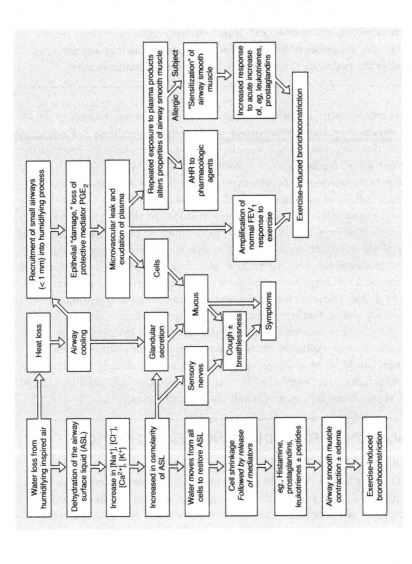

FIGURE 4.1 Flow chart describing the acute events leading to exercise-induced bronchoconstriction in the classic asthmatic (left) and the events leading to the development of exercise-induced bronchoconstriction in the athlete (right).

Source: Anderson, S. D. & Kippelen, P. 2005. Exercise-induced bronchoconstriction: pathogenesis. *Curr Allergy Asthma Rep*, 5, 116–122.

chemokines and growth factors) could, over time, modify the contractile properties of the muscle and increase airway responsiveness (Figure 4.1).

One way of explaining the reason for a very high prevalence of EIB in athletes is to consider that in athletes who train daily, chronic exposure of the airway smooth muscle to the many biologically active agents present in the plasma (such as cytokines, chemokines and growth factors) could, over time, modify the contractile properties of the muscle and increase airway responsiveness. In many ways the pathological process could be viewed as akin to an injury.

In atopic athletes with higher than normal levels of circulating immunoglobin E (IgE), the repeated cycles of injury-repair of the airway epithelium is thought to create an *in vivo* model of 'passive sensitisation' that potentiates the effects of the bronchoconstrictive mediators (i.e. histamine, PGD_2 and cysLTs) on airway smooth muscle, favouring the development of EIB (Figure 4.1). In elite summer-sport athletes, the risk of asthma – or so-called 'atopic asthma' – has been shown to increase with the number of positive skin test reactions to airborne allergens.

In winter-sport athletes, airway epithelial injury could be responsible for the high prevalence of 'ski asthma' or 'sports asthma' (i.e. asthma symptomatology and AHR, in the absence of allergic features). Severe heat and water losses during exercise in cold environments could, through airway epithelial injury and/or sensory nerves activation, stimulate cough and mucus production (i.e. the two most common symptoms reported by cross-country skiers). Further, injury to the airway epithelium (with shedding of epithelial cells) may facilitate access of pharmacological agents to receptors on the airway smooth muscle, thereby explaining the high proportion of skiers positive to methacholine challenge. Finally, repeated injury-repair of the airway epithelium would contribute to airway remodelling, with mucosal infiltration of inflammatory cells and thickening of the basement membrane (as observed in elite cross-country skiers;).

APPLICATION OF SCIENTIFIC PRINCIPLES TO PRACTICE

Given the increased prevalence of EIB in endurance, winter and pool-based sports (and to a lesser extent, stop and go sports), health professionals, coaches and support staff working with these categories of athletes should be particularly cognisant of the problem and how to reliably assess and treat this condition. They should recognise that it is not only athletes with clinical asthma who are at risk for EIB, and that systematic screening may be required in some athletic groups.

How should you diagnose EIB in athletes?

To optimally treat and manage EIB in athletes (with or without asthma), the first step is to diagnose the condition properly (see Chapter 5). Due to the poor sensitivity and specificity of symptoms to predict EIB, the role of respiratory symptoms in diagnosing EIB in athletes is minimal. Furthermore, while pulmonary function tests are the obvious first choice for the identification of EIB, athletes often have supra-normal basal lung function and spirometry results that may appear normal, despite the presence of airway abnormalities. Therefore, bronchial provocation tests are recommended for EIB diagnosis in athletes.

The progressive advancement in our understanding of the pathophysiology of EIB over the last fifty years has led to the development of various bronchial provocation tests that induce bronchoconstriction *via* different mechanisms. Indirect tests, including exercise, eucapnic voluntary hyperpnoea (EVH) of dry air and osmotic challenges (e.g. mannitol and hypertonic saline), initiate the release of mediators from inflammatory cells within the airways that cause the airway smooth to contract; as such, they closely mimic the real-life events triggered by exercise and are appropriate for the diagnosis of EIB (see Chapter 5). On the contrary, direct tests (e.g. methacholine) that act directly on specific airway smooth muscle receptors do not provide information about airway inflammation and are not recommended for EIB diagnosis.

Can you measure airway inflammation and airway injury?

Fractional exhaled nitric oxide (FeNO) is a marker of steroid-responsive inflammation that is commonly used in clinical practice to assess non-invasively airway inflammation, diagnose asthma and monitor adherence to therapy. While airway inflammation can be present in some athletes with EIB, neutrophilic and mixed inflammatory patterns have also been reported. Eosinophilia is not a prerequisite for EIB in athletes; therefore, FeNO is a poor predictor of EIB in athletic populations (Table 4.2). Nonetheless, in athletes under pharmacological treatment for asthma/EIB, a high FeNO may suggest suboptimal control and should prompt clinicians to revisit pharmacological options, inhalation technique and adherence to therapy.

Bronchial biopsies and induced sputum are more direct approaches to demonstrate airway inflammation and injury. However the complexity and invasiveness of these techniques renders them difficult to use in athletes (hence, seldom experimental data based on bronchial biopsies and sputum analyses) and preclude them from being routinely implemented in clinical practice (Table 4.2). A non-invasive alternative is the measurement of the club cell secretory protein-16 (CC16) in urine or serum. CC16 is a pneumoprotein secreted by the non-ciliated epithelial club cells; thus, predominantly localised to the peripheral airways. Increased leakage of CC16 in the bloodstream and a rise in urinary excretion of CC16 have been reported after strenuous exercise and dry air hyperpnoea in athletes, supporting the role of high ventilation in inducing airway epithelial injury. That the CC16 increase in urine is blunted and bronchoconstriction blocked when the exercise is

TABLE 4.2 Pros and cons of various biomarkers of airway inflammation/injury

Test	Marker of	Pros	Cons
FeNO	Eosinophilic inflammation	Non invasive Simple to administer Can be used for follow-up investigations (i.e. repeated measurements) Immediate results Published reference values Relatively low cost	Poor predictor of EIB Influenced by environmental and dietary factors Does not detect presence of alternative inflammatory profiles (e.g. neutrophilic inflammation)
CC16 in serum or urine	Airway epithelial injury	Minimally/non invasive Evaluation of peripheral airways Can be used for follow-up (i.e. repeated measurements)	High variability (influenced by many factors, incl. changes in glomerular permeability during exercise) Adjustment of serum values for the permeability of the alveolo-capillary barrier recommended (i.e. CC16/SP-D ratio) Requires immediate storage or analysis No published reference values Moderate cost
Induced sputum	Airway inflammation	Minimally invasive Characterisation of the type of inflammation (i.e. eosinophilic, neutrophilic, mixed) Published reference values	Necessitate high degree of cooperation Evaluation of central airways Possible contamination with nasal or pharyngeal secretions Wash-out period required for repeated measurements Moderate cost
Bronchial biopsies	Airway inflammation Airway remodelling	Direct assessment Characterisation of the type of inflammation	Invasive Highly skilled procedure Wash-out period required for repeated measurements Evaluation of proximal airways No published reference values High cost

FeNO, fractional exhaled nitric oxide; CC16, club cell secretory protein-16; SP-D, surfactant-associated protein D.

performed in warm humid air further suggests that warm humid air breathing is beneficial, not only to prevent EIB, but also to limit the degree of injury to the airways. Thus, wherever possible, athletes should be recommended to exercise in warm humid environments.

Exposure to pollutants (e.g. ozone) and irritants (e.g. chlorine) during exercise has also been shown to result in an increased urinary excretion of CC16. This result is consistent with our knowledge of an increased prevalence of EIB in athletes routinely exposed to polluted and chlorinated environments. It also supports the recommendation for athletes to limit exposure to noxious airborne agents when training.

At present, CC16 appears an interesting biomarker of airway epithelial injury, which could help identify strategies to protect the airways of athletes. However, heterogeneity of measurement renders interpretation of cross-sectional data difficult (Table 4.2). The biomarker may therefore be most useful in randomised controlled trials, where changes from baseline can represent acute injury to the airway epithelium.

How can you treat airway inflammation and injury?

As EIB is a disorder involving inflammation of the airways, inhaled corticosteroids (ICS) are the mainstay of treatment for EIB in athletes (Chapter 6). ICS are recommended for the treatment of 'atopic asthma' (characterised by allergic sensitisation, rhinitis and other allergic comorbidities and signs of eosinophilic inflammation) in athletes, since it shares many similarities to the classic presentation of asthma. Yet, ICS should not be prescribed to those athletes suffering from 'sports asthma'. In athletes with 'sports asthma' (incl. 'ski asthma'), the sole positive response to methacholine challenge is usually indicative of airway epithelial injury (not EIB), and is commonly associated with neutrophilic infiltration and airway remodelling; as such, ICS have demonstrated limited efficacy in the treatment of 'ski asthma'. The treatment of EIB is covered in Chapter 6.

CASE STUDY

Medical history: A 30-year-old male international long-distance triathlete was reporting mild symptoms of cough and mucus hyper-secretion during exercise, yet had no personal or family history of asthma or of EIB.

Examination: Baseline spirometry was normal: forced vital capacity (FVC) 5.36 L (107% pred.); forced expiratory volume in one second (FEV_1) 3.98 L (97% pred.); and FEV_1/FVC 74%. He performed two exercise challenges (i.e., 8-min runs near maximal aerobic capacity, with no warm-up) in warm humid (25°C, 86% relative humidity) and cold dry (4°C, 61% relative humidity) air on separate days. He reached ventilation rates >120 L min^{-1} (>80% of pred. maximum voluntary ventilation) on both occasions. In the warm humid environment, no significant change in FEV_1 was noticed after the challenge (FEV_1 Δ 5% of baseline). However, with the inhalation of cold dry air during exercise, a maximal fall in FEV_1 of 21% was recorded at 10 min post-challenge. The bronchoconstriction was sustained over 60 min and reversed by inhalation of 200 µg of Salbutamol. A skin prick test revealed significant atopy to grass. The athlete was diagnosed with EIB.

Management and outcome: The athlete was prescribed daily preventive treatment (i.e. corticosteroid by inhalation), and a long-acting β_2-agonist to be taken as needed before prolonged training session and/or competitions. After a year of treatment, his bronchial response to exercise normalised, with a maximum fall in FEV$_1$ post-challenge in cold dry air <10%.

Discussion: Screening for EIB is recommended in elite endurance sports. Inspiring cold air during exercise challenges enhances the possibility of EIB, thereby reducing false-negative diagnoses.

Conclusion

Athletes with and without clinical asthma who engage in endurance, winter or pool-based activities are at high risk for EIB. The physiological stimulus for EIB is the loss of water (by evaporation) from the airway surface when ventilatory demand increases. This loss of water causes transient dehydration of the small airways, epithelial injury and inflammatory mediator release. In athletes with EIB, the released mediators stimulate airway smooth muscle, causing its contraction and airway narrowing. Indirect bronchial provocation tests that trigger an inflammatory response in the airways and medications that treat the root of the problem (i.e. airway inflammation) should be used for the diagnosis and treatment, respectively, of EIB in athletes.

Summary

1. The prevalence of EIB varies considerably across sports, with athletes from endurance disciplines, swimmers and winter athletes particularly at risk.
2. Athletes with and without asthma may have EIB, with many athletes developing the condition 'late' in their career (at age 20 years or over).
3. The physiological stimulus for EIB is evaporative water loss from the surface of the airways when large quantities of unconditioned air are inhaled over a short period.
4. The water loss within the airways during strenuous exercise leads to airway cooling and dehydration, thereby triggering an inflammatory response and airway epithelial injury.
5. As EIB has an inflammatory basis, indirect bronchial provocation tests are preferred over direct tests for EIB diagnosis in athletes, and anti-inflammatory medications should be the cornerstone of EIB treatment.

Multiple-choice questions

For each question multiple answers may be correct.

1. Identify athletes at an increased risk for asthma/EIB:

    (A) Cyclists
    (B) Sprinters
    (C) Ice-hockey players
    (D) Cross country skiers
    (E) Ski jumpers

2. Which of the following factors is the key determinant of EIB in athletes?

(A) Heat loss within the upper airways
(B) Heat loss within the lower airways
(C) Water loss within the central airways
(D) Water loss within the small airways

3. According to the 'osmotic theory' of EIB, which cells get predominantly activated when the airway surface lining gets dehydrated by exercise-hyperpnoea:

(A) Macrophages
(B) Neutrophils
(C) Mast cells
(D) Lymphocytes

4. 'Ski asthma' is characterised by:

(A) Respiratory symptoms
(B) EIB
(C) Airway hyperresponsiveness to methacholine
(D) Airway remodelling
(E) Airway inflammation

5. Which of the following can be used as biomarker of airway epithelial injury?

(A) Fractional exhaled nitric oxide (FeNO)
(B) Serum level of eosinophil cationic protein (ECP)
(C) Sputum eosinophilia
(D) Urine level of club cell secretory protein-16 (CC16)

Key reading

Anderson, S. D. & Daviskas, E. 2000. The mechanism of exercise-induced asthma is … *J Allergy Clin Immunol*, 106, 453–459.

Anderson, S. D. & Kippelen, P. 2005. Exercise-induced bronchoconstriction: pathogenesis. *Curr Allergy Asthma Rep*, 5, 116–122.

Anderson, S. D., Sue-Chu, M., Perry, C. P., Gratziou, C., Kippelen, P., McKenzie, D. C., Beck, K. C. & Fitch, K. D. 2006. Bronchial challenges in athletes applying to inhale a beta2-agonist at the 2004 Summer Olympics. *J Allergy Clin Immunol*, 117, 767–773.

Bolger, C., Tufvesson, E., Anderson, S. D., Devereux, G., Ayres, J. G., Bjermer, L., Sue-Chu, M. & Kippelen, P. 2011. Effect of inspired air conditions on exercise-induced bronchoconstriction and urinary CC16 levels in athletes. *J Appl Physiol (1985)*, 111, 1059–1065.

Fitch, K. D. 2012. An overview of asthma and airway hyper-responsiveness in Olympic athletes. *Br J Sports Med*, 46, 413–416.

Fitch, K. D., Sue-Chu, M., Anderson, S. D., Boulet, L. P., Hancox, R. J., McKenzie, D. C., Backer, V., Rundell, K. W., Alonso, J. M., Kippelen, P., Cummiskey, J. M., Garnier, A. & Ljungqvist, A. 2008. Asthma and the elite athlete: summary of the International Olympic Committee's consensus conference, Lausanne, Switzerland, January 22–24, 2008. *J Allergy Clin Immunol*, 122, 254–260.

Helenius, I. J., Tikkanen, H. O., Sarna, S. & Haahtela, T. 1998. Asthma and increased bronchial responsiveness in elite athletes: atopy and sport event as risk factors. *J Allergy Clin Immunol*, 101, 646–652.

Karjalainen, E. M., Laitinen, A., Sue-Chu, M., Altraja, A., Bjermer, L. & Laitinen, L. A. 2000. Evidence of airway inflammation and remodeling in ski athletes with and without bronchial hyperresponsiveness to methacholine. *Am J Respir Crit Care Med*, 161, 2086–2091.

McFadden, E. R. 1990. Hypothesis: exercise-induced asthma as a vascular phenomenon. *Lancet*, 335, 880–883.

Rundell, K. W., Anderson, S. D., Sue-Chu, M., Bougault, V. & Boulet, L. P. 2015. Air quality and temperature effects on exercise-induced bronchoconstriction. *Compr Physiol*, 5, 579–610.

Rundell, K. W., Im, J., Mayers, L. B., Wilber, R. L., Szmedra, L. & Schmitz, H. R. 2001. Self-reported symptoms and exercise-induced asthma in the elite athlete. *Med Sci Sports Exerc*, 33, 208–213.

Simpson, A. J., Bood, J. R., Anderson, S. D., Romer, L. M., Dahlén, B., Dahlén, S. E. & Kippelen, P. 2016. A standard, single dose of inhaled terbutaline attenuates hyperpnea-induced bronchoconstriction and mast cell activation in athletes. *J Appl Physiol (1985)*, 120, 1011–1017.

Answers: 1 (A, C, D), 2 (D), 3 (C), 4 (A,C,D,E), 5 (D)

5

DIAGNOSIS OF EXERCISE-INDUCED BRONCHOCONSTRICTION

Oliver J. Price, John W. Dickinson and John D. Brannan

Overview

This chapter will cover:

- Respiratory symptoms (e.g. cough, wheeze, breathlessness etc.) are poorly predictive of the presence and/or severity of EIB in athletes.
- Objective clinical assessment via indirect bronchoprovocation testing is therefore required to confirm a diagnosis before initiating treatment.
- Exercise testing can have variable diagnostic sensitivity depending on the ambient environmental conditions and the protocol employed which presents a potential for misdiagnosis.
- Surrogate airway challenges such as EVH and inhaled mannitol are therefore currently recommended to confirm or refute a diagnosis.
- Indirect bronchoprovocation challenge tests also have utility in assessing efficacy to therapeutic interventions (i.e. inhaled corticosteroid therapy) prescribed to manage EIB.

Introduction

As discussed in Chapter 4, exercise-induced bronchoconstriction (EIB), in the presence or absence of clinical asthma, is the most prevalent chronic condition in athletic populations. Irrespective of the athletic standard or level of competition, securing a robust diagnosis of EIB is important in order to optimise and manage airway health, and in turn minimise the potential impact on sports performance. It is therefore important that sports physicians and applied scientists, who provide support or encounter athletes reporting troublesome exertional respiratory symptoms have a comprehensive understanding and appreciation of the challenges associated with diagnosis before initiating treatment. This is particularly relevant when applied to elite athletes (i.e. national and international standard) competing under the constraints of the World Anti-Doping Agency (WADA) Code, given several well-established pharmacological inhaler therapies are either prohibited in and out of competition and/or have a maximum permitted dose (see Chapter 6).

This chapter evaluates the current available diagnostic methodology for EIB and provides practical recommendations concerning clinical assessment, diagnostic test selection and interpretation.

Should respiratory symptoms be used in isolation to diagnose EIB?

It is common for athletes to report respiratory symptoms during high-intensity exercise, however due to distinguishing features often considered 'typical asthma symptoms' (e.g. cough, wheeze, breathlessness etc.) athletes who describe breathing difficulty are often prescribed an efficacy trial of inhaler therapy (e.g. salbutamol) for a presumed diagnosis of EIB. Although this approach may seem intuitive, a wealth of scientific literature opposes this practice due to the poor agreement between perceived respiratory symptoms and objective evidence of EIB in athletes. Indeed, the (in)accuracy of self-reported symptoms has previously been demonstrated to be imprecise at best, and at worst, no better than a coin-toss.

NOT ALL WHEEZE IS EXERCISE INDUCED BRONCHOCONSTRICTION (EIB)

The disparity between self-report respiratory symptoms and confirmation of EIB is complex and multifaceted. Respiratory symptoms should not be used in isolation to confirm a diagnosis for the following reasons:

1. A significant proportion of athletes with EIB do not perceive or complain of breathing difficulty during exercise and therefore remain undetected unless widespread screening interventions are implemented.
2. The under recognition of other prevalent and overlooked differential causes of exertional breathlessness in athletes remains a concern. For example, exercise-induced laryngeal obstruction (EILO) – a condition characterised by transient closure of the laryngeal inlet (voice box) during high-intensity exercise mimics asthma symptoms – thus presenting a potential for misdiagnosis (see Chapter 9). It is equally important to consider (and rule out) other forms of cardio-pulmonary disease, dysfunctional breathing patterns and/or physical deconditioning that present with breathlessness during peak exercise and improve with recovery.
3. Symptom perception is generally non-specific and personality trait and expectation of sports performance may influence the accuracy of a symptom-based diagnosis. It is also possible that athletes with pre-existing clinical asthma may under report symptoms due to dampened perception, which has been associated with long-term inhaled corticosteroid therapy.

The limited value of symptoms in this context is underlined by a recent qualitative study investigating the perception of breathing in athletes where very few
features helped to distinguish between EIB and non-EIB forms of breathlessness.
Although history of symptoms (i.e. exercise mode and intensity, sporting
environment, anatomical location, recovery time post exercise and response to
β_2-agonist therapy) should be considered during clinical assessment, objective
testing is required to minimise the risk of misdiagnosis (i.e. under or over-detec-
tion) and should therefore always be sought to confirm or refute a diagnosis.

Which objective airway challenge should I use to diagnose EIB?

As discussed in Chapter 4, the airway response to the dehydrating effects of hyperpnoea with sustained exercise causes the endogenous release of a variety of broncho-
constricting mediators that in susceptible individuals act on specific receptors that cause
the airway smooth muscle to contract. Diagnostic tests that induce bronchoconstriction via this mechanism are referred to as indirect bronchoprovocation challenges.

Airway inflammation is an essential component underlying the mechanisms
leading to airway narrowing. Indirect bronchoprovocation tests promote activation
of this pathway, which is why indirect airway challenges are now endorsed as the
optimal approach to confirm underlying EIB pathophysiology and identify individuals whom are likely to benefit from regular inhaled corticosteroid therapy.

This is in contrast to direct airway challenges that are most useful in the context
of determining whether an individual's symptoms are arising from current clinical
asthma. Direct challenges reflect the effect of only a single agonist or mediator (e.g.
methacholine or histamine) and have been reported to provide both low sensitivity
and specificity to detect EIB in athletic populations reporting symptoms. Although
an athlete presenting with a positive test outcome following a direct challenge,
current active respiratory symptoms, demonstrated airway reversibility with spirometry, and/or has other markers of airway inflammation (e.g. heightened fractional
exhaled nitric oxide and/or sputum eosinophils) will likely have EIB, an indirect
bronchoprovocation challenge is recommended to confirm a diagnosis in those
without pre-existing clinical asthma (Table 5.1). The following section will evaluate diagnostic protocols, procedures and techniques employed in clinical practice.

What instructions should be given to an athlete before an indirect bronchoprovocation test?

To standardise repeat assessment and monitor response to inhaler therapy, it is
important that athletes adhere to pre-test instructions closely prior to undergoing
an indirect bronchoprovocation challenge. Athletes should avoid treatments known
to be effective at attenuating or inhibiting EIB over the recommended washout
period prior to testing (i.e. anti-inflammatories, anti-histamines, short and long-
acting β_2-agonists and inhaled corticosteroids) and should be encouraged not to

TABLE 5.1 EIB diagnostic test selection

Diagnostic test	Strength in diagnosis	Rationale
Indirect bronchoprovocation		
Athletes with EIB & clinical asthma		
Sensitivity	✓✓✓✓	Both exercise and surrogate tests act via a similar mechanism to identify active inflammation and a sensitive airway smooth muscle.
Specificity	✓✓✓✓	A negative test indicates absence of active inflammation and a sensitive airway smooth muscle decreasing the likelihood of false-positive tests.
Athletes with EIB only		
Sensitivity	✓✓✓	For some individuals a second and sometimes third indirect test is warranted to exclude EIB with confidence.
Specificity	✓✓✓✓	Specificity remains high even in mild EIB.
Direct bronchoprovocation		
Athletes with EIB & clinical asthma		
Sensitivity	✓✓	Sensitivity is not high in those with newly diagnosed asthma with EIB or in athletes. Good lung function may protect AHR to a direct stimulus. Sensitivity increases when lung function is transiently reduced by inflammation or is persistent due to airway remodelling.
Specificity	✓✓	Specificity may decrease with increased likelihood of remodelling and reduced lung function, independently of inflammation causing EIB.
Athletes with EIB only		
Sensitivity	✓✓	Sensitivity is not as high as previously thought in athletes. Good lung function may protect AHR to a direct stimulus.
Specificity	✓✓	Specificity may decrease with increased likelihood of remodelling (e.g. winter sport athletes and airway damage due to chronic dehydration).

AHR: airway hyperresponsiveness; EIB: Exercise-induced bronchoconstriction.

perform vigorous exercise or ingest caffeine on the day of the test (refrain for at least 4 hours prior to the test). Furthermore, athletes should avoid wearing tight restrictive clothing to ensure chest wall mechanics are not impeded during pulmonary function manoeuvres (Table 5.2).

TABLE 5.2 Pre-test instructions for indirect bronchoprovocation challenge testing in athletes

Medication, exercise and diet	*Time to withhold prior to test*
Short-acting β_2-agonist (Albuterol, Terbutaline)	8 hr
Long-acting β_2-agonist (Salmeterol, Formoterol)	24 hr
Long-acting β_2-agonist in combination with an inhaled corticosteroid (Salmeterol/Fluticasone, Formoterol/Budesonide)	24 hr
Ultra-long acting β_2-agonists (Indacaterol, Olodaterol, Vilanterol)	≥72 hr
Inhaled corticosteroid (Budesonide, Fluticasone propionate, Beclomethasone)	6 hr
Long-acting inhaled corticosteroid (Gluticasone furoate)	24 hr
Leukotriene receptor antagonists (Montelukast, Zafirlukast)	4 days
Leukotriene synthesis inhibitors (Zileuton / Slow release zileuton)	12 hr / 16 hr
Anti-histamines (Loratadine, Citirzine, Fexofenadine)	72 hr
Short-acting muscarinic acetylcholine antagonist (Ipratropium bromide)	12 hr
Long-acting muscarinic acetylcholine antagonist (Tiotropium bromide, Aclidinium bromide, Glycopyrronium)	≥72 hr
Cromones (Sodium cromoglycate, Nedocromil sodium)	4 hr
Xanthines (Theophylline)	24 hr
Caffeine	24 hr
Vigorous exercise	>4 hr

Source: adapted from Weiler et al. (2016)

How do I undertake an exercise challenge?

Laboratory exercise challenge testing should be conducted as described in the consensus statements published by the American Thoracic Society (ATS), European Respiratory Society (ERS) and American Academy of Allergy, Asthma and Immunology (AAAAI).

When conducting an exercise challenge, the minute ventilation and water content of inspired air should be controlled as the achieved ventilation is key to providing the maximal provocative dehydrating stimulus to the airways. Exercise ramp-up must be rapid to reach a heart rate of ≥85% of maximum for adults and up to 95% for children within 2–3 minutes. It is recommended that exercise should continue at this rate for an additional 6 minutes while breathing dry air (e.g. medical grade supplied via a Douglas bag and a 2-way non-rebreathing valve) to achieve at least 40% of maximum voluntary ventilation (MVV) (calculated: 17.5 × baseline FEV_1). However, exercise ventilation ideally should be ≥60% of predicted MVV (calculated: 21 × baseline FEV_1) sto minimise false-negative outcome resulting from a sub-maximal stimulus. Minute ventilation of expired air should be measured in real-time using a high flow spirometer or metabolic cart.

Prior to exercise challenge, and at pre-determined times post exercise (3, 5, 7, 10 and up to 30 minutes post challenge) spirometry should be performed in accordance with international guidelines. However, a measurement at 1 minute post exercise may be warranted in athletes suspected of having bronchospasm during exercise, which may be evidenced by declines in minute ventilation and the presence of symptoms. All spirometry measures to determine FEV_1 should be performed seated and with full forced vital capacity (FVC) manoeuvres at the post-exercise time-points. EIB may be diagnosed by ≥10% fall in FEV_1 from the pre-exercise value at any two consecutive time-points within 30 minutes of exercise cessation. A fall at only one time-point may be considered diagnostic of EIB if a greater fall in FEV_1 is observed (i.e. ≥20% fall in FEV_1 required in pharmaceutical studies).

To determine whether the fall is sustained and not the product of a single measurement that may represent an artefact due to inadequate spirometry effort at one or more time-points, the profile of the fall in FEV_1 following exercise should be carefully examined. In mild bronchial hyper-responsiveness (BHR), it is important to note that there may be variability in the airway response to exercise when more than one test is performed and the results are compared. Thus, in some cases where EIB is strongly suspected or when the athlete is treated optimally and evidence of the abolition of EIB is required, repeat assessment may need to be considered.

Laboratory exercise challenge by treadmill is more easily standardised and more commonly performed in a hospital or human physiology laboratory setting. Alternative exercise challenges using cycle or rowing ergometers may be performed to align with the athlete's sporting discipline. However, compared to a treadmill challenge, cycle exercise may provide a sub-optimal ventilatory stimulus (i.e. lower ventilatory demand and humidity of ambient laboratory). To counter these issues, field-based and free running challenge tests have been proposed as an option and employed in the context of screening large groups of athletes (e.g. sports teams or squads). While this approach improves ecological validity, it is difficult to standardise the cardiovascular workload and ambient conditions of the environment when employing this approach and thus presents difficulties in both documenting and guaranteeing an optimal exercise intensity and dehydrating airway stimulus.

What constitutes a positive response on challenge testing?

Despite sport governing bodies requiring specific cut-off values to diagnose EIB, there is currently no single absolute cut-off for a fall in FEV_1 or change in other spirometry parameters that clearly and unequivocally distinguishes between the presence or absence of EIB. For elite athletes applying for a therapeutic use exemption to use otherwise banned asthma therapy (e.g. inhaled terbutaline), evidence of a sustained reduction in lung function is required to confirm a diagnosis (i.e. ≥10% fall in FEV_1 at two consecutive time-points).

The ATS criteria suggest the post-exercise fall in FEV_1 required to make a diagnosis must be at least 10%, whereas other groups have suggested a fall of 13% to 15% is necessary to rule-in a diagnosis. In contrast, other recommendations also include a fall in FEV_1 of 15% after a 'field' challenge and a fall of 6% to 10% in the laboratory. Due to the aforementioned challenges associated with establishing a secure diagnosis when employing exercise testing, several indirect surrogate tests have been developed in an attempt to overcome these limitations.

Can I use a surrogate test to diagnose EIB?

Organisations that regulate drug use by elite athletes or professional bodies (i.e. WADA) who are required to assess the presence of EIB by occupation are increasingly recommending the use of surrogate challenges for exercise such as EVH or the inhaled hyperosmolar agent inhaled mannitol. While EVH is a challenge test that should be used for the investigation of EIB alone, inhaled mannitol may be useful in identifying both EIB and the presence of clinical asthma.

How do I undertake an eucapnic voluntary hyperpnoea challenge?

The eucapnic voluntary hyperpnoea (EVH) challenge was developed on the premise that the ventilation reached and sustained, and the water content of the air inspired, are the most important determinants of EIB. When performing the EVH test, the athlete voluntarily hyperventilates a source of dry air containing approximately 5% carbon dioxide (CO_2) to maintain eucapnia, with the remainder of the gas mixture containing 21% oxygen and the balance nitrogen (74%). The athlete's maximum level of ventilation can be reached more rapidly with voluntary hyperventilation, reducing the required time for the EVH test in comparison to the exercise challenge. EVH has been observed to identify more cases of EIB than laboratory exercise tests, and it is as sensitive as field-based exercise testing for athletes. This is likely due to the higher levels of ventilation that can be rapidly achieved and sustained using EVH compared with laboratory exercise on a bicycle or treadmill.

While there are a number of different methods for EVH, a standardised single stage protocol involving inhaling a pre-prepared gas mixture for 6 minutes is most commonly employed. The required apparatus can be easily sourced and the initial set-up is relatively inexpensive compared with exercise challenge equipment. Commercial systems now exist permitting breath-by-breath delivery of dry air with the addition of CO_2 (Eucapsys system: www.smtec.net/en/products/eucapsys).

Real-time measurement of ventilation is recommended requiring a large meteorological balloon or a Douglas bag as a gas reservoir filled with at least 90 L of the dry air mixture containing 5% CO_2 (Figure 5.1). The athlete hyperventilates the air mixture via a two-way valve, keeping the balloon at a constant volume, while the gas from the cylinder refills the reservoir via a rotameter at the pre-calculated target ventilation of ≥60% MVV. The recommended ventilation is 30 times the baseline FEV_1 and it has been demonstrated that the majority of athletes are able to achieve this target. If the minimum ventilation is not reached, however, the test may be invalid and need repeating on a separate occasion. Following the period of ventilation, FEV_1 should be measured in duplicate at 3, 5, 7, 10, 15, 20 (and if required 30 minutes).

Is EVH testing safe and what constitutes a positive response?

For those with established clinical asthma frequently require β_2-agonists to alleviate respiratory symptoms, the EVH test should be performed with caution knowing that the airway stimulus is highly potent and therefore may induce significant bronchospasm in susceptible individuals. Thus, safety precautions should be implemented during an EVH test and should only be performed by trained specialists familiar with the procedure (e.g. respiratory physiologist or technician). The EVH test should not be performed on athletes in whom baseline FEV_1 is less than 75% of predicted. BHR may occur during ventilation and any sudden falls in

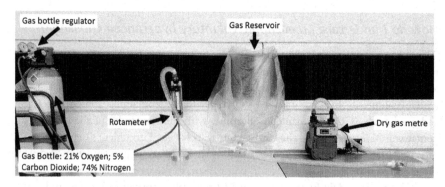

FIGURE 5.1 Eucapnic voluntary hyperpnoea challenge equipment set-up.

ventilation rate could be an indication of bronchoconstriction. In this scenario, the test may need to be terminated and FEV_1 measured immediately, followed by the administration of a rescue bronchodilator (i.e. 4 × 100ug salbutamol via pressurised metered dose inhaler and spacer).

A fall in FEV_1 ≥10% from the pre-challenge value is defined as a positive test and the severity of the fall in FEV_1 defines the severity of the BHR. It is recommended that the fall in FEV_1 should be sustained, with the subject having ≥10% fall in FEV_1 recorded at two consecutive time-points post challenge.

Can I use the FEV_1 fall following an exercise or EVH challenge to categorise EIB severity?

Severity of disease to exercise and EVH can be graded as **mild** if the FEV_1 fall from baseline following exercise or EVH challenge is ≥10–25%; **moderate** if the FEV_1 fall from baseline following exercise or EVH challenge is ≥25%-50%; or **severe** if the FEV_1 fall from baseline following exercise or EVH challenge is ≥50%.

How do I undertake an inhaled mannitol challenge?

The mannitol challenge test was developed to make an indirect challenge more clinically accessible to overcome the disadvantages of nebulisation and move beyond the hospital laboratory in order to be performed safely in a clinical setting. Inhaled mannitol, commercially available as a disposable kit (Aridol or Osmohale) (www.aridol. info) has been investigated for safety and efficacy and is a regulatory authority registered test in Australia, United States, European Union, Korea, and other regions.

Following reproducible baseline spirometry, the mannitol test requires the athlete to inhale increasing doses of dry powder mannitol and have the FEV_1 measured in duplicate 60 seconds after each dose step. The FEV_1 should be repeatable within 5%. The test protocol consists of 0-mg (empty capsule), 5mg, 10mg, 20mg, 40mg, 80mg (2x40mg capsules), and three dose steps of 160mg (4x40mg capsules) of mannitol. A positive test result is defined as either a fall in FEV_1 of 15% from baseline (i.e. post 0-mg capsule) or a 10% fall in FEV_1 from baseline between two consecutive doses. If an athlete presenting with symptoms suggestive of EIB has a fall ≥10% and <15% following the maximum cumulative dose of 635mg (i.e. only documenting a PD_{10}) then mild EIB could be considered. In some cases with very mild responses, validation may be useful by repeating the test or via an alternative indirect challenge (e.g. EVH).

The mannitol test needs to be performed in a timely manner without delay so that the osmotic gradient is increased with each dose. The time to complete a positive test as observed in a large Phase 3 trial was 17 minutes (±7 minutes) for a positive test, and 26 minutes (±6 minutes) for a negative test. Importantly, it was also found that test duration over 35 minutes may lead to a false-negative result. Coughing to mannitol may occur suggesting clinically relevant cough hypersensitivity. Inhaled mannitol has demonstrated safety both in established Phase 3 trials as well as in the field in epidemiology studies and shown to possess good reproducibility in asthmatic athletes.

Airway responses are reversed rapidly with a standard dose of bronchodilator. The airway sensitivity to mannitol strongly correlates with the % fall in FEV_1 to exercise in steroid naïve asthmatics. Mannitol has also been shown to identify BHR 1.4 times more than a 10% fall in FEV_1 to laboratory running exercise and 1.65 times more if a 15% fall to exercise is considered as an abnormal response in patients with newly diagnosed asthma. Further, mannitol is also more sensitive at identifying BHR compared to a laboratory cycle exercise in known asthmatic individuals. A summary of indirect bronchoprovocation challenge tests are provided in Table 5.3.

SUPPLEMENTARY DIAGNOSTIC METHODS

Due to the aforementioned challenges associated with securing a diagnosis of EIB – several adjunct tests are available to aid clinical decision-making:

1. **Impulse or forced oscillometry** is a non-effort dependent pulmonary function test designed to assess airway mechanics via random pressure pulses superimposed over tidal breathing. Although valid cut-off values have yet to be established, it has been proposed that impulse oscillometry may offer utility as a supplementary test to confirm or refute a diagnosis of EIB.
2. **Skin prick testing** may be a useful predictive tool aid the diagnostic work-up of EIB due to the strong association between atopy and severity of BHR in athletes. Testing should only be conducted by trained personnel in accordance with established international guidance.
3. **Fractional exhaled nitric oxide (FeNO)** is an indirect marker of airway inflammation. Raised FeNO (>50 ppb) has therefore been proposed to provide value in detecting EIB and monitoring the response to inhaled corticosteroid therapy.

How do I apply these assessments in real life practice?

It is important to employ a systematic approach to clinical assessment and diagnostic work-up, yet at the same time, consider athlete history concerning respiratory symptoms on an individual basis. It is recognised that adopting structured closed questions often considered important when assessing individuals with clinical asthma (e.g. 'Is your breathing worse in cold weather' or 'Do you wheeze or cough?') offer limited diagnostic value in the context of EIB. Employing a pragmatic consultation style and simply listening to the athlete 'story' or adopting a framework of open-ended questions designed to explore athlete symptoms (e.g. 'How would you describe your sensation of breathing during exercise?' or 'Describe a time when your breathing has been problematic during exercise') has been proposed to have greater value and may yield diagnostically useful information. Furthermore, requesting an audio or video recording when respiratory symptoms present during exercise (particularly in primary care) is a novel cost-effective approach that may confirm a sign of respiratory dysfunction (e.g. wheeze,

TABLE 5.3 Indirect bronchoprovocation challenges

Diagnostic challenge	Diagnostic criteria	Pros	Cons
Laboratory exercise challenge	$\geq 10\%$ fall in FEV_1 from baseline post exercise at two consecutive time-points A fall at only one time-point may be considered diagnostic of EIB if a significant reduction in lung function is observed (i.e. $\geq 20\%$ fall in FEV_1 required in pharmaceutical studies)	Standardised/controlled environment Exercise equipment inexpensive	Environment not sufficiently provocative for EIB in some athletes Failure to replicate physical demands / mode of sport Low diagnostic sensitivity Athlete may not comply with high intensity exercise requirement of the challenge
Laboratory exercise challenge (+ dry gas inhalant)	$\geq 10\%$ fall in FEV_1 from baseline post exercise at two consecutive time-points A fall at only one time-point may be considered diagnostic of EIB if a significant reduction in lung function is observed (i.e. $\geq 20\%$ fall in FEV_1 required in pharmaceutical studies)	Controlled environment Controlled dry gas inhalant – higher diagnostic sensitivity than ambient atmospheric air No requirement to transport testing equipment to field based setting	Increased routine cost of test (dry air) Dry air environment not representative of athlete training environment Athlete may not comply with high intensity exercise requirement of the challenge
Field-based exercise challenge	$\geq 10\%$ fall in FEV_1 from baseline post exercise at two consecutive time-points A fall at only one time-point may be considered diagnostic of EIB if a significant reduction in lung function is observed (i.e. $\geq 20\%$ fall in FEV_1 required in pharmaceutical studies)	Sports specific Transportable equipment	Unable to control environment and cardiovascular workload Low diagnostic sensitivity

(Continued)

Table 5.3 (Cont.)

Diagnostic challenge	Diagnostic criteria	Pros	Cons
Eucapnic voluntary hyperpnoea	$\geq 10\%$ fall in FEV_1 from baseline post EVH at two consecutive time-points	High diagnostic sensitivity Controlled dry gas inhalant Improved ability to maximise and sustain minute ventilation in well-trained athletes	Not sports specific Consumable costs of running test greater than exercise Dry air environment not representative of athlete training environment Specialised gas required for test (21% O_2, 5% CO_2, balance N_2)
Mannitol challenge	Either a fall in FEV_1 of 15% from baseline (i.e. post 0-mg capsule) or a 10% fall in FEV_1 from baseline between two consecutive doses. If an athlete presenting with symptoms suggestive of EIB has a fall $\geq 10\%$ and $<15\%$ following the maximum cumulative dose of 635mg (i.e. only documenting a PD_{10}) then mild EIB could be considered	Controlled dose-response test Portable equipment	Not sports specific Low diagnostic sensitivity (particularly in winter sport-based athletes)

stridor, laboured breathing or cough) to support clinical suspicion or inform referral for specialist testing.

Training athletes to use portable lung function equipment (i.e. spirometers and/ or peak expiratory flow metres) may also provide value in a field-based setting, or long-term surveillance of airway health / response to therapy. Caution is clearly advised when adopting this approach and should not be used to confirm or refute a diagnosis or replace clinical assessment (i.e. indirect bronchoprovocation testing) conducted by trained personnel.

Following consultation, baseline spirometry should be performed and evaluated for evidence of expiratory airflow obstruction (i.e. FEV_1/FVC <0.7). If detected, a bronchodilator reversibility challenge should be conducted to confirm or refute a diagnosis of clinical asthma (≥12% increase in FEV_1) which would suggest an increased risk of EIB; particularly in patients with greater severity (reversible) expiratory airflow limitation at rest. In contrast, in the scenario baseline spirometry values are within normal predicted limits, test selection should focus on indirect bronchoprovocation. Due to the aforementioned limitations associated with exercise testing, surrogate challenges (i.e. EVH or inhaled mannitol) should be conducted in the first instance with post challenge spirometry used to confirm or refute a diagnosis. If a negative EVH or mannitol test is confirmed in a symptomatic athlete (i.e. EIB ruled-out with confidence), referral for differential diagnosis should be considered (Figure 5.2; also see Chapters 8–11).

Can I use indirect airway challenges to monitor response to EIB therapy?

Indirect bronchoprovocation challenges also provide value in the investigation of drugs employed to treat clinical asthma and EIB. Furthermore, pharmacotherapy effective in attenuating EIB has been shown to inhibit the airway response to both EVH and mannitol. Indeed, when treatment is optimal, it is thought to be possible to abolish BHR to these stimuli and thus minimise the potential negative impact of BHR on exercise performance.

Current guidelines recommend the regular use of an inhaled corticosteroid to treat EIB, particularly in cases where acute inhibition using β_2-agonist therapy is persistent and due to concerns that regular high-dose β_2-agonist therapy is associated with β_2-receptor tolerance (i.e. reduced efficacy over time). Repeat assessment or surveillance of EIB using exercise or a surrogate test provides valuable information concerning the optimal treatment effects of regular inhaled corticosteroid therapy or potential lack of efficacy in the presence of regular β_2-agonist administration. This may be important considering there are no known genetic sub-types to predict resistance to the effects of regular β_2-agonists on EIB.

Studies investigating inhaled corticosteroid therapy have demonstrated that higher doses appear to be more effective at inhibiting EIB when treatment is initially introduced. In contrast, studies evaluating long-term therapy have reported that when administered daily, lower inhaled corticosteroid doses may be equally as

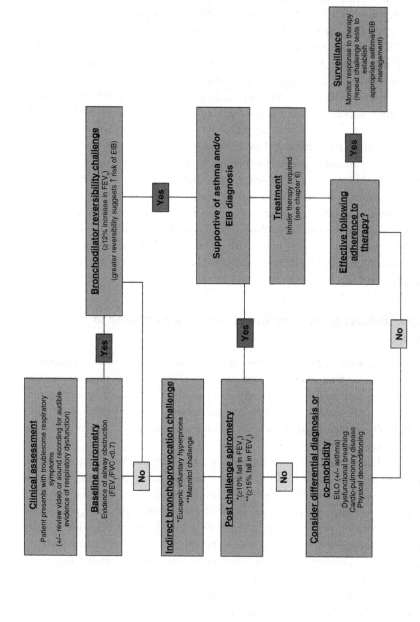

FIGURE 5.2 Diagnostic algorithm to confirm or refute exercise-induced bronchoconstriction in athletes.

effective. Indeed, following short-term use of inhaled corticosteroids, improvements in EIB have been associated with a reduction in sputum eosinophils. Asthmatics with higher levels of eosinophils appear to have the greatest immediate benefit when prescribed a higher dose of inhaled corticosteroid. Although sputum eosinophils have been shown to diminish significantly following only 3-weeks of inhaled corticosteroid therapy, EIB may still be present, indicating that the number and activity of mast cells (a key cell implicated in the mechanism of EIB), may take longer to reduce following inhaled corticosteroid treatment. Considering this, more rapid attenuation of EIB can occur in those with milder EIB. Accordingly, athletes with more severe EIB likely have greater airway inflammation and therefore may require longer surveillance, where ongoing monitoring may justify the requirement for longer-term adherence therapy. To date, there are no studies to suggest that regular pharmacotherapy other than inhaled corticosteroid therapy can effectively attenuate EIB over the long-term. However, at the elite level of sport, it may be preferable to objectively assess the efficacy of more than one acute therapy to determine if combination treatment provides more complete attenuation of EIB. This approach is particularly relevant given the inter-individual variation in treatment responses observed using pharmacotherapeutic agents in the treatment of clinical asthma and EIB (see Chapter 6).

Clinical case study examples

Scenario 1

25-year-old recreational level male triathlete with no prior history of asthma presents with troublesome respiratory symptoms including cough, wheeze and breathlessness that occur during and up to 15 minutes post exercise.

Diagnostic work-up

Evaluation of respiratory symptoms during consultation and objective assessment of baseline airway inflammation (FeNO). Spirometry conducted before and following an EVH challenge.

Clinical outcome

Normal baseline lung function within predicted limits. Normal resting FeNO (14ppb). 11% fall in FEV_1 at one time-point post challenge indicates borderline (mild severity) EIB. Consider either repeat assessment or alternative challenge (e.g. exercise or mannitol) before initiating therapy to confirm or refute a diagnosis of EIB before initiating treatment. Consider differential diagnose of dysfunctional breathing or exercise induced laryngeal obstruction.

Scenario 2

31-year-old male elite level swimmer reports breathing difficulty during periods of high volume/intensity training.

Diagnostic work-up

Evaluation of respiratory symptoms during consultation and objective assessment of baseline airway inflammation via FeNO. Spirometry conducted before and following an EVH challenge.

Clinical outcome

Normal baseline lung function within predicted limits. Elevated resting FeNO (43ppb) and 35% fall in FEV_1 from baseline following EVH challenge confirms moderate EIB. Inhaled corticosteroid therapy prescribed daily and adherence encouraged. Short acting β_2-agonist recommended before exercise. To confirm efficacy of inhaled corticosteroid, EVH was re-assessed at 3-months permitting the re-evaluation of pre-exercise β_2-agonist. Athlete reported that they had failed to adhere to prescribed inhaler therapy during the 3 month period. The repeat EVH challenge at 3-months demonstrated resting FeNO (45ppb) and a 50% reduction in the post EVH challenge fall in FEV_1. Further education and adherence to inhaler therapy was offered and encouraged. A follow-up 6 months after the initial EVH challenge identified the athlete was now adhering to inhaler therapy and reports of breathing difficulty in the pool were barely present and not impacting on training. FeNO 6 months after the initial EVH challenge had fallen to 22 ppb. The EVH challenge conducted 6 months after the initial challenge, resulted in an FEV_1 fall of 8% from baseline. The athlete's EIB now appears well managed and they are encouraged to maintain inhaler therapy.

Scenario 3

17-year-old female recreational runner presents with upper respiratory symptoms including tightness around throat and a high-pitch inspiratory 'whistling' during peak exercise. Current β_2-agonist reliever inhaler medication reported to provide limited value.

Diagnostic work-up

Evaluation of symptoms during consultation and objective assessment of airway inflammation (FeNO). Spirometry was conducted pre-and-post EVH challenge.

Clinical outcome

Normal baseline lung function within predicted limits. Normal resting FeNO (10ppb). 5% fall in FEV_1 reduction in lung function confirms a negative test result for EIB. Achieved ventilation during the test <60% predicted consistent with upper airway closure during exercise. Due to the persistence and nature of the symptoms, the athlete was referred for a continuous laryngoscopy during exercise test to confirm EILO. If high-symptom burden continues following EILO therapy (see Chapters 12 and 13), consider repeat EVH assessment to confirm or rule-out co-existing EIB.

Scenario 4

24-year-old elite 800 m runner presents with tight chest, excess mucus production, expiratory wheeze and breathing difficulty only when exercising in pollen environment.

Diagnostic work-up

Evaluation of symptoms during consultation and objective assessment of airway inflammation (FeNO). Spirometry was conducted pre-and-post EVH challenge.

Clinical outcome

Normal baseline lung function within predicted limits. Elevated resting FeNO (65 ppb) and 8% fall in FEV_1 from baseline following EVH challenge. Athlete achieved >60% MVV during EVH challenge. Decision made to conduct a field based exercise challenge outside at the athletes training venue during high pollen count. At follow-up athlete had a normal baseline lung function and elevated FeNO (62 ppb). The fall in FEV_1 post exercise challenge was 18% fall in FEV_1 confirming mild EIB in high pollen environment. Inhaled corticosteroid therapy prescribed daily and adherence encouraged. Short acting β_2-agonist recommended before exercise. Repeat exercise challenge the following year in high pollen environment resulted in reduced FeNO (23 ppb) and max fall in FEV_1 post exercise of 2%.

Conclusion

To optimise the care afforded to athletes reporting exertional respiratory symptoms, objective clinical assessment via indirect bronchoprovocation testing is required to confirm a diagnosis before initiating treatment – and EVH or inhaled mannitol are recommended for this purpose. Following a robust diagnosis, surveillance of airway health and monitoring the response to therapy (i.e. follow-up repeat objective assessment of EIB) is recommended to optimise management. In contrast, in the context of a negative diagnosis where EIB has been ruled-out with confidence, it is important to keep in mind that 'not all wheeze is EIB' and that a broad differential diagnosis (and potential for co-morbidity) exists in young athletes reporting breathing difficulty.

Multiple-choice questions

1. Exercise-induced bronchoconstriction is the term to describe:

    (A) Upper airway closure during vigorous exercise
    (B) Temporary expiratory airflow limitation in association with vigorous exercise
    (C) Respiratory symptoms during and post exercise
    (D) Breathing difficulty during exercise in people living with asthma

2. The key determinant(s) of exercise-induced bronchoconstriction are:

    (A) The intensity of exercise
    (B) The duration of exercise
    (C) The water content of inspired air
    (D) All of the above

3. Indirect bronchoprovocation challenges act to cause airway narrowing by:

    (A) Causing airway cooling that leads to smooth muscle contraction
    (B) Simulating the dehydrating mechanism hyperpnoea that has a direct effect on airway smooth muscle contraction
    (C) Acting via specific IgE mechanisms
    (D) Increasing airway osmolarity that cause mast cell degranulation and bronchoconstricting mediator release that has a direct effect on airway smooth muscle contraction

4. In the absence of an exercise test to confirm EIB, the most sensitive outcome that predicts EIB severity is:

    (A) Bronchodilator reversibility testing
    (B) Respiratory symptoms suggestive of EIB
    (C) Fraction of exhaled nitric oxide test
    (D) A surrogate indirect bronchial provocation test

5. A positive test result for EIB is most commonly defined using which pre-to-post diagnostic threshold:

    (A) $\geq 20\%$ fall in FEV_1

(B)   ≥10% fall in FEV_1
(C)   ≥15% fall in FEV_1
(D)   ≥25% fall in FEV_1

Online resources

How to perform an EVH test: www.youtube.com/watch?v=3U6y9AwDRN0.

Key reading

Anderson, S. D. 2010. Indirect challenge tests: Airway hyperresponsiveness in asthma: its measurement and clinical significance. *Chest*, 138, 25S–30S.

Brannan, J. D. 2010. Bronchial hyperresponsiveness in the assessment of asthma control: Airway hyperresponsiveness in asthma: its measurement and clinical significance. *Chest*, 138, 11S–17S.

Brannan, J. D., Koskela, H., Anderson, S. D. & Chew, N. 1998. Responsiveness to mannitol in asthmatic subjects with exercise-and hyperventilation-induced asthma. *American Journal of Respiratory and Critical Care Medicine*, 158, 1120–1126.

Dickinson, J. W., Whyte, G., Mcconnell, A. & Harries, M. 2006. Screening elite winter athletes for exercise induced asthma: a comparison of three challenge methods. *British Journal of Sports Medicine*, 40, 179–182.

Graham, B. L, Steenbruggen, I., Miller, M. R., Barjaktarevic, I. Z., Cooper, B. G., Hall, G. L., Hallstrand, T. S., Kaminsky, D. A., McCarthy, K., McCormack, M. C., Oropez, C. E., Rosenfeld, M., Stanojevic, S., Swanney, M. P. & Thompson, B. R. 2019. Standardization of Spirometry 2019 Update. An Official American Thoracic Society and European Respiratory Society Technical Statement. *American Journal of Respiratory and Critical Care Medicine*, 200, e70–e88.

Hallstrand, T. S., Leuppi, J. D., Joos, G., Hall, G. L., Carlsen, K.-H., Kaminsky, D. A., Coates, A. L., Cockcroft, D. W., Culver, B. H. & Diamant, Z. 2018. ERS technical standard on bronchial challenge testing: pathophysiology and methodology of indirect airway challenge testing. *European Respiratory Journal*, 52, 1801033.

Hull, J. H., Ansley, L., Price, O. J., Dickinson, J. W. & Bonini, M. 2016. Eucapnic voluntary hyperpnea: gold standard for diagnosing exercise-induced bronchoconstriction in athletes? *Sports Medicine*, 46, 1083–1093.

Miller, M. R., Hankinson, J., Brusasco, V., Burgos, F., Casaburi, R., Coates, A., Crapo, R., Enright, P. V., Van Der Grinten, C. & Gustafsson, P. 2005. Standardisation of spirometry. *European Respiratory Journal*, 26, 319–338.

Parsons, J. P., Hallstrand, T. S., Mastronarde, J. G., Kaminsky, D. A., Rundell, K. W., Hull, J. H., Storms, W. W., Weiler, J. M., Cheek, F. M., Wilson, K. C. & Anderson, S. D. 2013. An official American Thoracic Society clinical practice guideline: exercise-induced bronchoconstriction. *American Journal of Respiratory Critical Care Medicine*, 187, 1016–1027.

Price, O. J., Ansley, L., Levai, I. K., Molphy, J., Cullinan, P., Dickinson, J. W. & Hull, J. H. 2016a. Eucapnic voluntary hyperpnea testing in asymptomatic athletes. *American Journal of Respiratory and Critical Care Medicine*, 193, 1178–1180.

Price, O. J., Hull, J. H., Ansley, L., Thomas, M. & Eyles, C. 2016b. Exercise-induced bronchoconstriction in athletes–a qualitative assessment of symptom perception. *Respiratory Medicine*, 120, 36–43.

Rundell, K. W., Im, J., Mayers, L. B., Wilber, R. L., Szmedra, L. & Schmitz, H. R. 2001. Self-reported symptoms and exercise-induced asthma in the elite athlete. *Medicine and Science in Sports and Exercise*, 33, 208–213.

Weiler, J. M., Brannan, J. D., Randolph, C. C., Hallstrand, T. S., Parsons, J., Silvers, W., Storms, W., Zeiger, J., Bernstein, D. I., Blessing-Moore, J., Greenhawt, M., Khan, D., Lang, D., Nicklas, R. A., Oppenheimer, J., Portnoy, J. M., Schuller, D. E., Tilles, S. A. & Wallace, D. 2016. Exercise-induced bronchoconstriction update-2016. *J Allergy Clin Immunol*, 138, 1292–1295.

Answers: 1 (B), 2 (D), 3 (D), 4 (D), 5 (B)

6

PHARMACOLOGICAL TREATMENT OF ASTHMA-RELATED ISSUES IN ATHLETES

Matteo Bonini and James H. Hull

Overview

This chapter will cover:

- The medical treatment of asthma and exercise induced bronchoconstriction.
- Consider the implications of treatment for athlete health.
- Ensure that any inhaler therapy prescribed is utilised in a logical way and inhaler technique is checked.
- Discuss the implications of any treatment with respect to anti-doping regulations.
- How to approach emergency treatment.

Introduction

An understanding of the best approach to the pharmacological treatment of asthma and EIB is vital to any clinician wishing to optimise respiratory care in athletes. Indeed, if asthma +/− EIB is treated correctly then an athlete's symptoms should be completely ameliorated and thus the aim of treatment is to ensure that the affected athlete reports no problems while undertaking sport. This is a fact borne out by published data that reveals that asthmatic athletes, when treated appropriately, outperform their non-asthmatic counterparts in Olympic competition; despite a substantial literature base indicating that asthma medications, when taken at a regular prescribed dose, confer no ergogenic benefits. Thus, the fact that an athlete is asthmatic should never be used to deter them from aiming for the top step of the podium (Figure 6.1).

Generally speaking, the approach to treating an athlete with asthma should align with international asthma guidance statements, such as that produced by the global initiative for asthma (GINA – see https://ginasthma.org). This guidance is constantly updated and certainly within the past five years the pharmacological approach to asthma management

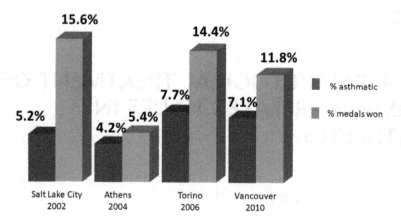

FIGURE 6.1 Percentage of athletes with asthma using inhaled β₂-agonists therapy at Summer and Winter Olympic Games and the percentage of medals won by those athletes.
Source: adapted from Fitch (2012)

has evolved significantly. Specifically, there has been increased availability and use of biologic treatments to target the underlying immunological derangements apparent in the asthma process (e.g. use of anti–IL-5 treatment). In addition, there have been randomised control studies indicating that an 'as needed' approach to treatment may work for many individuals, providing it is utilised with an inhaled corticosteroid component (i.e. as needed use of budesonide-formoterol combination).

There are however a number of important considerations that need taking into account in when treating athletes; not least, the concerns regarding the impact of side effects, regularity of use with a risk of tachyphylaxis and anti-doping regulations. It is thus recommended that more specific or athlete-focussed guidance is sought, when available (see further reading). While this chapter aims to offer an overview of treatment approach and to act to highlight some key points to consider, it is recommended clinicians should access online guidance, to get the most up to date recommendations and thus to remain truly informed on contemporary practice. Moreover, while many clinicians often feel comfortable prescribing inhalers, it is our experience that very few spend time discussing and reviewing inhaler technique or ensuring good medication adherence.

The aim of this chapter is to cover these issues, but to also highlight that while pharmacological treatment is considered the mainstay of asthma management, it is probably best viewed and prescribed in conjunction with non-pharmacological strategies (see Chapter 7).

What is the first-line approach to treatment?

Short-acting β₂-agonist (SABA) inhaled treatment (e.g. salbutamol, albuterol or ter-butaline) or the 'blue inhaler' has been long established as the standard first line treatment for athletes with asthma +/− EIB. This is not without good reason; when given in an inhaled dose (10–15 minutes pre-exercise) or with intermittent administration before exercise, SABA has been found to be the most effective drug to prevent the fall in FEV_1 that occurs during exercise; providing complete protection against exercise (FEV_1 fall <10%) in approx. 70% of subjects. The effect usually lasts 2h to 4h for SABA and up to 12h for long acting β_2-agonist (LABA).

However, there is evidence of heterogeneity in the observed efficacy of β_2-adrenergic agents to prevent EIB. This seems to be dependent not on the type of the molecule used, but rather on the population sample, with more variable effects reported in children. It also appears that chronic or long-term frequent use of SABA and/or LABA often results in a reduction of the duration and/or magnitude of protection against EIB, with cross-reacting tolerance to other β_2-agonists (i.e. at the time an athlete really needs bronchodilation, the inhaler will be less effective). This impaired efficacy has been shown to be predicted by baseline levels of FeNO (see Chapter 5). In fact, when subjects with EIB were grouped according to the recent ATS guideline recommendations for FeNO interpretation, those with values greater than 50 ppb showed a significantly higher loss of broncho-protection (LOB) with salmeterol against exercise, compared with those with values less than 25 ppb. Tolerance to β_2-agonists is only partially prevented by concomitant use of ICS.

Daily use of SABA and LABA may result even in a worsening of EIB and expose subjects to an increased risk of cardiovascular side-effects and death. Therefore, SABA and LABA should be used with caution on a regular basis to prevent EIB. LABA administration should also not be given without concomitant use of ICS according to the warning set by the US Food and Drug Administration.

MY INHALER ISN'T WORKING – WHAT NEXT DOC?

A point that is often overlooked is the fact that there is a significant minority (15–20%) of asthmatics whose EIB is not prevented by β_2-agonists, even when inhaled corticosteroids are used concomitantly. Thus, report of a 'lack of effi-cacy' when prescribing treatment to an asthmatic athlete should prompt con-sideration of the following questions:

i   Reconsideration of the diagnosis – was EIB objectively confirmed?
ii   Is the inhaler being taken correctly? Review and check inhaler technique.
iii   Is the inhaler being take regularly? Review and check prescription records – where does the athlete pick up their medication script from?
iv   Is there a co-existing problem (e.g. EILO and asthma together) that is masking any treatment response?
v   Could the athlete be resistant to the treatment? Check their provocation response while *on* treatment.

Is there a role for other types of reliever inhaler?

Ipratropium bromide can also be used, pre-exercise, to prevent EIB, although the effect is not consistent among patients and may be variable, even within the same patient. In the general asthma population, ipratropium lost favour against SABA treatment, given the more rapid action of SABA. Whether subjects with EIB without asthma or with a prevalent autonomic imbalance represent a phenotype more responsive to anticholinergic agents is an interesting hypothesis, still waiting for further experimental testing. Some studies, in fact, support the notion that athletes with high vagal tone may respond well to anti-cholinergics and indeed there is anecdotal evidence that this type of treatment may help athletes with overlapping EILO (see Chapter 9). The long-acting muscarinic agent Tiotropium could also be considered and is now licensed for asthma treatment in many countries.

Mast cell stabilisers, disodium cromoglycate and nedocromil sodium, attenuate both asthma and EIB when inhaled shortly before exercise. These agents have been shown to inhibit inflammatory mediator release and to reduce bronchoconstriction. However, the degree of broncho-protection afforded by cromones is lower than inhaled β_2-agonists (~50 *versus* ~66%, respectively) and their duration of action is relatively short (1–2 h).

Anti-inflammatory preventive drugs

The regular use of inhaled corticosteroid (ICS) is a key step for controlling the inflammatory processes that are present in the majority of individuals with asthma. Indeed, an overall increase in the use of ICS on a population level has been responsible for the steady reduction in asthma associated mortality seen over the past 30 years. Most guideline documents for many years have therefore highlighted the importance of regular ICS treatment in any asthmatic individual. This being said, more recently there is emerging evidence that indicates that in mild asthma, an 'as needed' approach to ICS/LABA treatment may be as effective as regular daily LABA/ICS approach.

More recently, several guidelines have advocated measurement of 'inflammatory' markers, sometime termed inflammometry, including techniques such as measurement of FeNO or sputum eosinophils, to help provide guidance on which individuals are more likely to respond favourable to ICS. This acknowledged, a number of studies have indicated that athletes with asthma may not demonstrate the classical inflammatory signal associated with ICS response (e.g. eosinophilia) and indeed some forms of 'sport' asthma are associated with inflammatory changes (i.e. a T2 low pattern) that are more generally deemed to be associated with a 'lack of ICS responsiveness'. Regardless, prophylactic administration of ICS is generally recommended for athletes, particularly if physical activity is performed regularly (>3 times per week), thus representing a repetitive stimulus for the onset of bronchoconstriction.

INHALED STEROID TREATMENT – HAVE THE CONVERSATION

In general, it is believed that ICS therapy is under-utilised in athletes. This may be partly because of the frequent lack of other features indicating steroid responsive clinical asthma in sport-related EIB (e.g. exacerbations, night waking) but may also relate to athlete and coach 'perceptions' of what 'steroid' means.

Many athletes are concerned that taking a 'steroid' inhaler may be misconceived as form of cheating and that there is something unnatural about taking this type of medication. It is thus vital that any clinician helping an athlete with asthma explains that ICS treatment does not enhance performance (i. e. that is why they are not prohibited by WADA) and that this treatment is important to prevent asthma and control the underlying process driving the problem.

Leukotriene antagonists (e.g. montelukast) have been reported to be effective in preventing EIB. However, protection appears to only occur in only approximately half of the subjects and may not be complete.

Are there any alternative or add-on medications?

The use of monoclonal antibodies or biologic treatment (i.e. anti-IgE, anti-IL5, anti-IL5r and anti-IL4r) has been proven to be effective and safe in asthma, however biologic based treatment is currently only utilised for individuals with severe disease (e.g. in the UK, mostly those dependent on regular oral corticosteroid or at least four courses per year and on maximal inhaler therapy).

Theophylline, calcium channel blockers, α-adrenergic receptor antagonists, inhaled furosemide, heparin, and hyaluronic acid have been studied to prevent EIB, but with inconsistent results and are thus not recommended for use by athletes.

What other factors should I consider when treating an asthmatic athlete?

A broad series of co-factors and drivers may influence the response to asthma treatments in athletes and should be therefore taken into high consideration.

Comorbidities also seem to play a relevant role in asthma prevalence and management. It has been in fact extensively reported that asthma and allergic rhinitis frequently coexist, with symptoms of rhinitis being reported in 80–90% of asthma patients, and asthma symptoms reported in 20–40% of patients with allergic rhinitis. Furthermore, it has been proven that the severity of allergic rhinitis and asthma is related and that proper management of allergic rhinitis improves asthma control. On the basis of the above, the Allergic Rhinitis and its Impact on Asthma (ARIA) recommendation to screen every subject with rhinitis for asthma should be also extended to athletes. The best treatment of any sino-nasal contribution is covered in Chapter 8.

Oral H1 antihistamines have for long been considered an effective therapeutic option for treating allergic rhinitis one of the most common asthma comorbidities, which has been shown to represent a significant and independent risk factor for the onset and worsening of asthma. However, these drugs may affect vigilance and reaction time in athletes, negatively impacting on their sport performances. The new generation molecules (i.e. cetirizine, desloratadine, fexofenadine, evocetirizine, loratadine, mizolastine) with higher selectivity and a longer half-life is preferable.

Reflux can also often co-exist with asthma and thus any athlete with 'airway-centric' type symptoms, such as cough or upper airway discomfort should complete a reflux specific airway questionnaire (e.g. the Hull airway reflux questionnaire) and be provided with treatment recommendations to tackle both acid (e.g. with a proton pump inhibitor) and non-acid (e.g. with Gaviscon) components of reflux.

Specific immunotherapy (SIT) biologically alters the immune response to allergens at early stages, thus resulting in diminished symptoms and need for drugs. Its efficacy has been proven for both rhinitis and asthma, and the association of the two diseases is the optimal indication. SIT must be prescribed and administered only by trained physicians, after a careful diagnostic and cost/benefit evaluation. There is no contraindication to immunotherapy in athletes. The only precaution should be to avoid physical exercise just after receiving the injection. Although the introduction of the sublingual administration has greatly increased the safety and practicality of this treatment, the use of immunotherapy is still currently limited in athletes.

How should I prescribe and check treatment?

It is our experience that athletes with a new diagnosis of asthma are often informed of the diagnosis, prescribed an inhaler and then essentially discharged to manage the condition on their own. Clearly this runs a real risk of suboptimal treatment and any athlete with a diagnosis of asthma should be afforded the best possible guidance and monitoring / surveillance to ensure the highest chance of therapeutic success.

In the general asthma population, it is well recognised that both inhaler technique and treatment adherence is suboptimal in the vast majority of patients. Patient adherence to prescribed treatment has been also shown to represent a crucial link between effective therapy and improved disease outcomes. However, several studies have revealed unsatisfactory compliance with guideline recommendations and a significant underuse of asthma therapy. Adherence to inhaled corticosteroids (ICSs) has been reported to be an independent strong predictor of long-term asthma control. A significant proportion of adult patients with difficult-to-control asthma showed poor adherence to corticosteroid therapy.

Appropriate inhalation technique is crucial for optimal delivery of drugs to the airways, despite it has been reported that most of asthma patients commit critical errors in inhaling manoeuvres. In our experience, many young athletic individuals tend to inhale at very high flow rates and thus prescribing a spacing chamber, can help to ensure that the correct flow rate is used.

CHECKING INHALER TECHNIQUE – WHY AND HOW

There is currently a great myriad of inhalers available on the marketplace. Many utilise different medication delivery systems and thus it is important that you spend time with the athlete discussing the use of their specific device and explain the steps involved in ensuring effective delivery.

1. Failure to use inhalers correctly reduces their efficacy.
2. Patients should be taught how to use their inhaler when they are first prescribed inhaled medication and not just given generic advice.
3. Their technique should be checked at subsequent consultations.
4. Individuals' abilities should be taken into account when selecting inhaler devices and in athletes it is often necessary to use a spacing device to ensure that they control the inspiratory flow rate.
5. Placebo inhalers can be useful to demonstrate correct inhaler technique.

What do I need to know about asthma treatment and anti-doping?

Doping, the use of prohibited drugs or methods to improve training and sporting results, remains one of the greatest problems of elite sport in the 21st century. Special precautions must be taken in competitive and professional athletes with regard to the World Anti-Doping Agency (WADA) rules on the use of anti-asthma medications. Elite athletes with asthma and their medical advisors must be aware of and always comply with the WADA Code and Prohibited List which is updated annually. An overview of the current (2020) asthma therapy position on the WADA Code and Prohibited List can be seen in Table 6.1.

All glucocorticoids (GC) are prohibited in competition when administered by systemic routes (i.e. intravenous, oral), while they are permitted if used as inhalers. Mast cell stabilisers, leukotriene antagonists and ipratropium bromide are no under restriction.

Although currently there is no evidence of a significant beneficial effect of inhaled β_2-agonists on physical performance when these medications are taken at therapeutic recommended doses (i.e. not abused at very high doses), these drugs are included in the WADA list of substances subject to limitations. This was following report of an anabolic effect on the cardiac and skeletal muscle exerted by albuterol and to the hypothesis that these drugs could mimic the effects produced by the endogenous catecholamines. Having said this, WADA has produced guidance allowing the use of some SABA and LABA, providing a certain threshold is not surpassed.

TABLE 6.1 2020 WADA anti-doping rules for anti-asthmatic drugs

Treatment	WADA rules	Notes
Antihistamines	Permitted	Second generation molecules should be preferred to avoid side effects
Leukotriene modifiers	Permitted	
Inhaled steroids	Permitted	
Immunotherapy	Permitted	SCIT should not be performed before or after physical exercise
β_2-agonists	Inhaled salbutamol: maximum 1600 mcg/24H in divided doses not to exceed 800mcg/12H Formoterol (max 54 mcg/24H) and Salmeterol (max 200 mcg/24H) All others prohibited in and out competition	The presence in urine of salbutamol in excess of 1000 ng/mL or formoterol in excess of 40 ng/mL is presumed not to be an intended therapeutic use of the substance and will be considered as an Adverse Analytical Finding
Systemic steroids	*Prohibited in competition*	
Ephedrine, methylephedrine	*Prohibited in competition*	A concentration in urine greater than 10 ug/ml represent an Adverse Analytical Finding

WHAT SHOULD I DO TO CHECK IF A MEDICATION IS PROHIBITED OR IN AN EMERGENCY?

For clear advice and guidance on this issue visit www.globaldro.com or call your respective national anti-doping organisation (e.g. UK Anti-doping).

If you are treating an athlete in an emergency – then document all the clinical features in a robust and clear way (e.g. including all clinical findings and investigations) and then approach treatment as you would any other individual (i.e. don't withhold treatment you would use routinely for fear of a future anti-doping infringement).

An athlete's health should never be compromised by withholding medication in an emergency.

What is a therapeutic use exemption (TUE)?

Some pharmacological treatments used for asthma require a therapeutic use exemption or TUE for short. The idea behind a TUE is that it allows an athlete to use a certain medication that is vital to maintain their health, but which has not been shown to do any more than to simply restore them to 'normal' health. This is contentious and some believe that TUEs should be abolished. Having said this, the

TUE process enables asthmatic athletes to be given treatments such as oral corticosteroid to treat a major exacerbation (if they are *in competition*) and is used to allow diabetic athletes to use insulin.

If a TUE is needed then there will be specific guidance on the relevant anti-doping website (e.g. UK Anti-doping) on how to apply for one. Following this the TUE is assessed by a TUE Committee (TUEC). To approve an application for a TUE the following criteria must be met:

1. The drug is necessary to treat an acute or chronic medical condition and the athlete would experience a significant impairment to health if it were to be withheld.
2. The therapeutic use of the prohibited drug is highly unlikely to produce any additional enhancement of performance beyond what might be anticipated by a return to the athlete's normal state of health following the treatment.
3. There is no reasonable permitted therapeutic alternative to the use of the prohibited drug.
4. The necessity to administer the prohibited drug is not a consequence of the prior misuse of a prohibited drug or method.

Conclusions

This chapter has provided an overview of some of the issues faced when considering the pharmacological treatment of asthma $+/-$ EIB in athletes. The principles used to treat asthma in the general population should be followed and international guideline documents adhered to. Any treatment that is initiated should be carefully prescribed with due consideration for delivery technique and subsequent adherence. Readers should consult some of the key sources of information below for further detail.

Multiple-choice questions

1. The following statements are true:

    (A) Asthma usually limits Olympic performance
    (B) Asthmatic athletes should be given larger doses of inhaler therapy than usually used, given large lung capacity
    (C) Inhaler technique check is not necessary in athletes given they are usually bright and technically aware
    (D) Inhaled corticosteroids are prohibited in athletes
    (E) Salbutamol is prohibited by WADA

2. The following are clinically appropriate treatment options to prevent EIB in athletes:

    (A) Short-acting β_2-agonists alone
    (B) Long-acting β_2-agonists alone
    (C) Anti-histamine tables

(D) Theophylline tablets

(E) All of the above

3. If an athlete presents with an acute asthma severe attack it is vital that you:

(A) Don't use oral steroid to treat, because it is prohibited

(B) Use more β_2-agonist but advise the athlete to drink water so as not to pass a urine threshold for the permitted amount

(C) Use a new biologic asthma treatment because they are not prohibited

(D) Ask them to consult their sports coach first to see if it is ok for them to have emergency asthma treatment

(E) Treat as per your usual practice but document all assessments and treatment carefully and consider the need for an athlete to apply for a TUE.

4. A therapeutic use exemption (TUE) is:

(A) A means of getting approval to use a sabultamol inhaler

(B) A document that proves an athlete has asthma

(C) Necessary for an athlete wishing to take inhaled steroid

(D) Allows an athlete to take as much inhaler as they wish

(E) Necessary for an athlete who is prescribed oral corticosteroid in competition.

5. In the treatment of asthma in an athlete it is important that you:

(A) Recognise and explain that no treatment is perfect and that the athlete should be realistic about their chances of making the Olympics.

(B) Provide at least two short acting β_2-agonist inhalers – in case an athlete needs to use a whole device before an important competition.

(C) Check inhaler technique, specific to the device prescribed

(D) B and C above

(E) none of the above

Online resources

Global DRO: www.globaldro.com

Global Initiative for Asthma: https://ginasthma.org

TUE β_2-agonist application form: www.ukad.org.uk/sites/default/files/2019-05/Beta-2%20Agonist%20TUE%20Application%20Form.pdf

WADA TUE application form: https://www.wada-ama.org/en/resources/therapeutic-use-exemption-tue/tue-application-form

Key reading

Fitch K. (2012). An overview of asthma and airway hyperresponsiveness in Olympic athletes. *Br J Sports Med*, 46, 413–416.

Fitch K. (2016). The World Anti-Doping Code: can you have asthma and still be an elite athlete? *Breathe*, 12, 148–158.

Parsons J, Hallstrand T, Mastronarde J, Kaminsky D, Rundell K, Hull J, Storms W, Weiler J, Cheek F, Wilson K & Anderson S. (2013). An official American Thoracic Society clinical practice guideline: exercise-induced bronchoconstriction. *Am J Respir Crit Care Med*, 187, 1016–1027.

Salpeter SR, Ormiston TM, Salpeter EE. (2004). Meta-analysis: respiratory tolerance to regular beta2-agonist use in patients with asthma. *Ann Intern Med*, 140(10), 802–813.

Weiler J, Brannan J, Randolph C, Hallstrand T, Parsons J, Silvers W, Storms W, Zeiger J, Bernstein D, Blessing-Moore J, Greenhawt M, Khan D, Lang D, Nicklas R, Oppenheimer J, Portnoy J, Schuller D, Tilles S & Wallace D. (2016). Exercise-induced bronchoconstriction update-2016. *J Allergy Clin Immunol*, 138, 1292–1295.

Answers: 1 (A), 2 (A), 3 (E), 4 (E), 5 (C)

7

NON-PHARMACOLOGICAL MANAGEMENT OF ASTHMA-RELATED ISSUES IN ATHLETES

Neil C. Williams, Michael A. Johnson, Emily M. Adamic and Timothy D. Mickleborough

Overview

This chapter will cover:

- Non-pharmacological management options for athletes with asthma and EIB.
- The benefit of high-intensity interval warm-up to reduce the severity of EIB in a subsequent exercise bout.
- The impact of dietary modification on EIB.
- The place for dietary supplementation with caffeine or omega-3 fish oils.
- The emerging evidence to indicate targeting the gut microbiota through dietary interventions of prebiotics as a potential adjunct treatment for EIB.

Introduction

As discussed in the previous chapter inhaled pharmacological therapy is the mainstay of EIB/asthma management. However, pharmacologic treatments are not curative and do not modify disease progression. Moreover, the use of certain inhalers may also be associated with adverse side effects and chronic use of β_2-agonists can induce tachyphylaxis (i.e. render them progressively less effective). Furthermore, athletes may not want to take medication or may not adhere to prescribed medication, which can result in poor asthma control and negative effects on exercise performance.

It is therefore important for athletes and coaches to be well informed and educated about the options for the management of asthma and EIB using non-pharmacologic approaches. The purpose of this chapter is to examine and describe the evidence regarding the efficacy and mechanism(s) of action of some non-pharmacologic approaches that may serve as adjunct therapies for asthma and EIB. We focus on whether the severity of EIB is attenuated by an appropriate pre-exercise warm-up or by wearing a heat exchanger facemask during exercise. Furthermore, dietary factors that can modulate the immune system and the pathogenesis of asthma and EIB will be examined; in particular, we describe the effects of reduced dietary salt intake, and supplementation with caffeine, fish oils (omega-3 poly-unsaturated fatty acids), prebiotics and probiotics.

Can a warm-up reduce the risk and severity of EIB?

Approximately half of individuals with EIB will experience a reduction in airway responsiveness during repeated exercise. This 'refractory period' can be advantageous to athletes if exploited in the correct way and therefore, athletes with EIB may consider performing a specific pre-exercise warm-up.

A high-intensity, intermittent exercise, which includes intensities close to maximal oxygen uptake or maximal heart rate, is suggested to be effective in reducing the fall in FEV_1 by approximately 11% after subsequent exercise. Indeed, in contrast to what may be expected a continuous exercise warm-up, performed at low- (60% maximal oxygen uptake or maximal heart rate) or high-intensity (close to maximal heart rate) is less effective at reducing EIB.

PRE-EXERCISE WARM-UP RECOMMENDATIONS

High-intensity intermittent exercise is effective in reducing the fall in FEV_1 after a subsequent exercise bout. A pre-exercise warm-up could consist of one of the following and be tailored to the individual athlete and subsequent exercise session.

- Two sets of 26 s sprints with 90 s recovery and a 5 min rest between sets.
- Eight maximum effort 30 s sprints with 45–90 s recovery between each sprint.
- Seven 30 s sprints at a speed equivalent of 120–130% of first sprint with 150 s recovery between each sprint.

The protective effect of warm-up exercise on EIB is attributed to a refractory period, which can last from 1 to 4 hours. Although the putative mechanisms underpinning the refractory period remain uncertain, it is likely due to receptor tachyphylaxis at the level of the airway smooth muscle to bronchoconstrictive mediators rather than their reduced release from mast cells.

Although an intermittent high-intensity warm-up may offer some protection against EIB, a caveat is that significant thermoregulatory strain and/or muscle metabolic perturbation elicited by the warm-up may compromise subsequent exercise performance. However, to avoid this problem, refractoriness can also be achieved using a specific respiratory warm-up comprising eucapnic voluntary hyperpnoea (EVH; see Chapter 5 for EVH set-up). In mild asthmatics with EIB, 10 minutes of EVH at intensities of 30–80% of maximal voluntary ventilation attenuated the fall in FEV_1 after a subsequent exercise challenge. The respiratory warm-up also reduced the perception of respiratory exertion during exercise and did not compromise exercise tolerance. Therefore, athletes could use a respiratory or high-intensity intermittent exercise warm-up to lessen the severity of EIB.

WHOLE BODY VERSUS RESPIRATORY WARM-UP

Whole body warm-up

Pros

- Sport specific.
- Whole body preparation for subsequent exercise.

Cons

- High-intensity exercise might not be appropriate for all athletes and exercise scenarios.
- High-intensity exercise may cause perturbations in the exercising muscles and compromise subsequent performance.

Respiratory warm-up

Pros

- Reduced risk of fatigue or injury prior to subsequent exercise bout.
- Once familiarised simple protocol to perform.

Cons

- Evidence of effectiveness in mild asthmatics only.
- Requires specialist equipment.
- Some athletes are not keen to perform EVH due to side effects such as coughing and dry throat.

Can a facemask help warm and moisten the air to reduce EIB severity?

Exercise in cold and dry environments can trigger EIB, especially when ventilation rates are high (see Chapter 4). To alleviate the impact of cold dry air on the airways, athletes can wear a heat and moisture exchanger (HME) facemask during exercise (Figure 7.1). These facemasks warm the inspired air and recover exhaled moisture, while adding minimal resistance to breathing even at high flow rates. When individuals with asthma wear a HME facemask during exercise in sub-freezing temperatures (around $-12°C$), the post exercise fall in FEV_1 is attenuated from approximately -30% to -13%. Whether regular use of a HME facemask has implications for airway inflammation and remodelling remains unknown. Furthermore, although a HME facemask is comfortable to wear under controlled

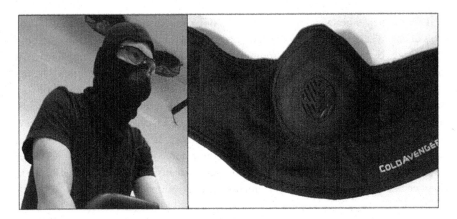

FIGURE 7.1 Athlete wearing a heat exchanger mask.

laboratory conditions, it might be cumbersome when worn during training and / or competition. Athletes should also ensure that using a HME facemask during competition falls within the rules of their sport's governing body. A list of UK sport governing bodies is accessible via Sport England (www.sportengland.org).

Can dietary salt modification reduce EIB severity?

High sodium intake was first linked to the prevalence and severity of asthma through epidemiological studies. As such, these findings have been extended to individuals with EIB.

High-salt diets (HSD) worsen and low salt diets improve pulmonary function and severity of EIB in a dose-dependent manner.

The sodium and chloride ions in dietary salt both play a role in airway reactivity. Reducing either sodium or chloride ions can ameliorate EIB, while reducing both can have an additive effect. While the precise mechanism is unknown, salt could act directly to increase bronchial smooth muscle tone and contractility via disruption of ion balance across the smooth muscle cell membrane. Alternatively, these ions could act indirectly by (1) increasing blood volume and thus pulmonary capillary volume, which increases airway compression and/or (2) increasing airway surface liquid osmolarity and hypertonicity, which induces the release of pro-inflammatory mediators such as leukotrienes and prostaglandins. These leukotrienes are responsible for the inflammatory response.

A low-salt diet (LSD) is typically defined as <1500 mg of sodium per day and an HSD as ~5000 mg/day. However, compliance to an LSD can be challenging and requires careful monitoring by coaches and/or support staff. This can be difficult when food labels often only display sodium and not chloride. To help compliance and provide incentive, athletes should be educated of the importance of maintaining an LSD for airway health. Templates for easy meal planning or comprehensive lists of high-sodium and low-sodium foods can be given to assist in athlete adherence. To measure progress, 24–hour urine tests can be done that quantify daily sodium excretion.

Despite their efficacy, adopting an LSD is not a feasible year-long solution. Proto-cols of two weeks LSD (~1500 mg sodium) have been found effective. Those that use only one week LSD (~1500 mg sodium) have been shown to be equally effective at ameliorating the drop in post exercise FEV_1 (peak fall in FEV_1 on normal salt diet −27% vs peak fall in FEV_1 one week of LSD −9%). Thus, this diet can be implemented during periods of high training stress or while training in cold or dry environments. LSDs can be used alone or in combination with other pharmacological and non-pharmacological strategies to manage airway reactivity. It is worthwhile to note that while effective against EIB, dietary salt intake may not alter resting airway function in asthmatic athletes. Additionally, there is limited evidence to support the relationship between salt intake and pulmonary function in non-asthmatics.

UTILITY OF LOW SALT DIETS FOR ATHLETES WITH EIB

High-salt diets can worsen EIB symptoms in two main ways: (1) increasing pulmonary capillary blood volume, causing airway compression, and/or (2) increasing osmolarity of the airway surface liquid which stimulates release of pro-inflammatory mediators, causing airway narrowing. Because of these effects, adoption of a low-salt diet can mitigate the severity of EIB in affected athletes by as much as a 27% (reduction in the fall in FEV_1 post-exercise). However, these diets are hard to maintain in common western cultures due to the salt content of common foods. As such, the use of LSD's may be most fea-sible during peak training or competition periods, and athletes should be assisted with food guides and meal plans to help promote adherence.

Can caffeine reduce EIB severity?

Caffeine is not currently on the World Anti-Doping Agency prohibited substance list, though it is part of a 'monitoring program'. Caffeine is chemically and pharmacologically related to the drug theophylline, which has anti-inflammatory, immunomodulatory, and bronchodilating effects. In adults with asthma, a caffeine dose of 10 mg·kg^{-1} consumed 1.5 hours before an EVH challenge reduced the fall in FEV_1 from 18% to 7%. Also in patients with asthma, a caffeine dose of 7 mg·kg^{-1} consumed 2 hours before 8 minutes of treadmill walking exercise at 85% maximum heart rate reduced the post-exercise fall in FEV_1 from 25% to 10%. In moderately trained recreational athletes, caffeine at 3, 6 and 9 mg·kg^{-1} consumed 1 hour before an incremental treadmill exercise test to exhaustion reduced the post-exercise fall in FEV_1 in a dose dependent manner from 18% to 12%, 9% and 7%, respectively. The 9 mg·kg^{-1} dose was also as effective in blunting EIB as a short acting β_2-agonist inhaler which is important because regular and frequent use of β_2-ago-nists can be associated with reduced protection against, and relief from, EIB. The empirical research is limited and has not specifically focussed on athletes; however, col-lectively the evidence suggests that caffeine consumption may offer some protection against EIB in a dose–response manner.

While the caffeine dose required to reduce EIB is markedly higher than typical dietary intakes, this dose is easily achieved if caffeine is taken in pill or powder form, which also allows close control of the consumed dose. This can be challenging when consuming caffeinated beverages such as coffee, which can have large variation in its caffeine content. Because the method of ingestion affects caffeine absorption rate, this should be considered with respect to timing of ingestion.

The benefits of consuming high doses of caffeine for protection against EIB must also be considered alongside the potential adverse side effects (increased heart rate, jitters), which in susceptible individuals may negatively affect exercise performance. Concerns regarding fluid-electrolyte imbalances due to caffeine-induced diuresis are, however, unwarranted.

Can fish oil supplementation impact EIB severity?

Airway inflammation, induced by pro-inflammatory mediators released in the airway, causes bronchoconstriction and compromises pulmonary function. To counter this, supplementation with fish oil has been used as a dietary means to manage airway inflammation and thus bronchial reactivity in asthmatic athletes. Fish oil can be consumed in the diet via fatty fish or supplementation with capsules, providing omega-3 (n-3) poly-unsaturated fatty acids (PUFAs) to the athlete.

Omega-3 PUFAs have been shown to reduce airway inflammation (measured by amount of pro-inflammatory leukotrienes in sputum) and severity of EIB (measured by post-exercise pulmonary function) in asthmatics or athletes who experience EIB.

PUFAs include both eicosapentaenoic acid (EPA) and docosahexaenoic acid (DHA), which are incorporated into the cell membrane of airway epithelial cells. It is here they exert their respective anti-inflammatory effects; EPA competes with arachidonic acid derivatives as a substrate for cyclooxygenase, blunting the production of pro-inflammatory leukotrienes. DHA may modify gene expression and signalling pathways related to inflammatory mediators such as tumour necrosis factor and heat shock proteins. EPA appears to be more effective than DHA in blocking eicosanoid and cytokine synthesis in human asthmatic alveolar macrophages, and in asthmatic humans DHA supplementation alone had no effect in mitigating EIB. Therefore, the ratio of EPA:DHA in fish oil supplements becomes an important consideration in any supplementation plan. Additionally, it is important to note that these protective effects are unique to n-3 PUFAs; n-6 PUFAs have opposite and deleterious effects, promoting pro-inflammatory leukotriene and prostanoid production.

MECHANISMS OF N-3 PUFAS

n-3 poly-unsaturated fatty acids (PUFAs) such as EPA and DHA are anti-inflammatory compounds that act on the airway epithelium, reducing the magnitude of the airway hyperactive response and thus mitigating the severity of exercise-induced bronchoconstriction. Supplementation as low as 1.8g EPA and 1.3g DHA per day with fish oil, over periods of 20 days or more, provides athletes with protective doses.

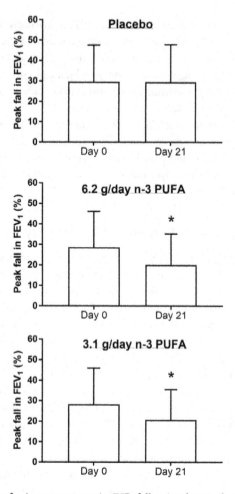

FIGURE 7.2 Evidence for improvements in EIB following lower doses of n3-PUFA.

The dose per day and the length of the supplementation period are two important variables when deciding upon an n-3 PUFA protocol. While doses of 3.2g EPA and 2.0g DHA per day have been shown to be effective, comparable improvements in EIB severity have been achieved using half those amounts (1.8g EPA and 1.3g DHA per day; see Figure 7.2). This is important, as low dose supplementation increases compliance, reduces cost and risk of gastrointestinal complaints. A supplementation period of 21 days is effective at reducing EIB severity regardless of dose. Alternatively periods of 30 days (3g per day) or as long as 12 months (84mg EPA per day) have been employed with success in different asthmatic populations. Fish oil could be used in combination with other asthma management strategies, although no additive effect was found with montelukast or vitamin C supplementation. Considering this, the overall strategy for asthma management must be carefully chosen on an individual basis for each athlete, using a combination of supplement protocols that are most effective for that person.

Can vitamins and antioxidants reduce EIB severity?

Oxidative stress is a clinical feature of EIB. Reactive oxygen species (ROS) and reactive nitrogen species (RNS) induce pro-inflammatory cell activation, increase mucus secretion, and increase airway hyperresponsiveness and inflammation. Dietary supplementation with antioxidants, primarily vitamins C (ascorbic acid) and/or E (α-tocopherol) may therefore benefit those with asthma and EIB, although limited research has been undertaken. Nevertheless, vitamin C supplementation (1500 mg/day for 2-weeks) in adults with mild-moderate asthma lowered the post-exercise fall in FEV_1 (−6%) compared with a usual (−14%) and placebo diet (−12%). This attenuation of EIB was associated with reduced intensity of asthma symptoms and lowered FeNO and urinary concentrations of pro-inflammatory mediators, which is indicative of reduced airway inflammation. Similarly, combined vitamin C (500 mg/day) and E (300 IU/day) supplementation for 2 weeks in adults with mild-moderate asthma also lowered the post-exercise fall in FEV_1 (−12%) compared with placebo (−20%). It is unknown if supplementation with both vitamins C and E provides greater protection against EIB than either vitamin alone. Furthermore, although antioxidant supplementation may reduce the severity of EIB, a caveat is that the dose required may blunt some of the skeletal muscle adaptations to strength and endurance training.

Can prebiotics and probiotics impact EIB severity?

The human body is home to trillions of symbiotic microorganisms (the microbiota) that colonise the skin, oral cavity, and the intestinal and respiratory tracts. The microbiota within the gut have a significant influence on immune function and may thereby influence airway health. This gut-lung axis thus represents a promising target for maintenance of airway health, and for the non-pharmacological management of asthma and other airway conditions. Beneficial changes in the gut microbiota can be achieved through dietary supplementation with probiotics (i.e. live microorganisms), prebiotics (i.e. non-digestible carbohydrates that increase the growth and activity of beneficial gut microbes such as the Lactobacillus and Bifidobacterium species), or both (i.e. synbiotic).

In murine models of allergic asthma, dietary prebiotics, probiotics and synbiotics have all been shown to reduce airway inflammation and improve disease severity. Initial investigations have shown positive effects of prebiotic supplementation in adults with asthma. Over a three week period, a daily dose of 5.5g of galactooligosaccharide (prebiotic) attenuated the FEV_1 fall post EVH challenge by 40% (−28 vs. −17%). Prebiotic supplementation reduced baseline serum markers of airway inflammation (CCL17 and C-reactive protein) and abolished the 29% increase in pro-inflammatory cytokine TNF-α after EVH.

Targeting the gut microbiota through prebiotic supplementation has the potential to modulate the underlying immunopathology of asthma, and thereby attenuate the airway hyperresponsiveness associated with EIB.

The mechanisms by which the gut microbiota influence asthma and EIB remain incompletely understood, but may include a contribution from: (I) short chain fatty acids that are produced by gut microbes fermenting prebiotics and soluble fibre, which affects immune function and inflammation; (II) dendritic cell sampling of the gut microbiota, which alters naïve T-cell differentiation towards a more beneficial T-regulatory profile; and (III) improvements in gut permeability and mucosal integrity which may influence systemic inflammation. Despite a current lack of mechanistic confirmation, there is growing evidence that prebiotics and probiotics could be a novel nutritional intervention to improve airway health and target EIB in physically active asthmatics. However, exact guidelines on dose and strain for probiotics are currently lacking.

PREBIOTIC AND EIB CASE STUDY SUCCESS

37-year-old (senior 4 age category) triathlete – diagnosed asthma and EIB – well controlled with baseline FEV$_1$ 90% predicted. Before treatment with 5.5g/d of prebiotic the athlete experienced a peak fall in FEV$_1$ of 47% after EVH. After 21 days of prebiotic supplementation (5.5 g per day) the athlete experienced a peak fall in FEV$_1$ of 17% EVH. This represents a dramatic 62% improvement in the peak fall in FEV$_1$ (Figure 7.3).

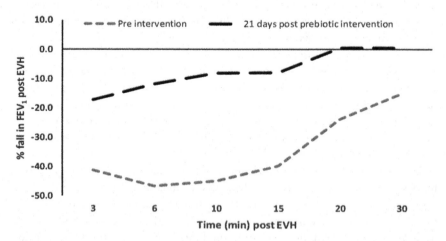

FIGURE 7.3 EVH challenge response before and following 21 days of prebiotic supplementation; demonstrating attenuation in the fall in FEV1 post-challenge.

HOW CAN ATHLETES MODIFY DIET TO REDUCE EIB?

- Athletes should aim to reduce dietary salt intake during periods of high training load, or when in an environment that triggers their asthma.
- Athletes with EIB should aim to increase their consumption of foods high in omega-3 polyunsaturated fatty acids. Examples include salmon, mackerel, and flax seeds.
- Increase consumption of gut microbiota friendly foods. This would include a higher dietary fibre intake (wholegrain, oats, barley), and increase consumption of fresh fruit and vegetables that can have a prebiotic effect (onions, artichoke, chicory, leeks, bananas).
- Increase consumption of foods high in antioxidants and polyphenols (berries and currants).

TABLE 7.1 Non-pharmacological strategies to manage EIB

Strategy	Intervention	Potential effect	Pitfalls
Pre-exercise warm-up	Repetitive 30-s bouts close to VO_{2max}/HR_{max}	Reduces EIB severity	May accumulate peripheral fatigue prior to exertion
Face masks	HME face masks	Reduces EIB severity	May affect ventilation and be associated with discomfort
Omega-3 fatty acid supplementation	3 g/d EPA and 2 g/d DHA	Reduces airway and systemic inflammation Reduces EIB severity	Side effects: Acid reflux, bloating, diarrhoea and nausea
Caffeine	5–10 mg/kgbw	Induces bronchodilation Reduces EIB severity Improves respiratory muscle fatigue resilience Counteracts exercise-induced hypoxaemia	Slow absorption Side effects: Muscle tremors, tachycardia
Vitamins and anti-oxidants	1500 mg/d vitamin C 64 mg/d β-carotene	Reduces systemic inflammation Reduces EIB severity	Side effects: diarrhoea, vomiting, headache, insomnia, nausea, kidney stones

Adapted from Dickinson et al. (2018)

Conclusion

Several non-pharmacologic strategies could contribute to the management of EIB in athletes. However, while some evidence supports the efficacy of some non-pharmacologic strategies, they should not replace prescribed pharmacological therapy. Rather, non-pharmacologic strategies should be considered as adjunct therapies that can supplement regular pharmaceutical therapy. Many studies have focused on non-athletes with EIB, thus more research is required to evaluate the effects of non-pharmacologic strategies in elite level athletes with EIB. The mechanistic pathways by which EIB is attenuated after different dietary interventions are likely to differ, but it remains unknown if the benefits of different interventions are additive. Therefore, further research is required to examine whether combined interventions are more effective at reducing EIB.

Multiple-choice questions

1. Which of the following is NOT an important consideration when choosing an omega-3 supplementation plan?

   (A)   Ratio of EPA/DHA
   (B)   Minimal effective dosage to avoid side effects
   (C)   Additive effects with other supplements
   (D)   Omega-3 vs. omega-6 PUFAs

2. Which of the following is a major barrier to low salt diets?

   (A)   Long restriction periods necessary for effectiveness
   (B)   High salt content in many people's natural diet
   (C)   Risk of side effects
   (D)   Lack of labelling on many food products

3. Which of the following is the correct definition of a dietary prebiotic?

   (A)   Dietary supplementation of live microorganisms to the gut
   (B)   Non-digestible carbohydrates that increase the growth and activity of beneficial microbes in the gut
   (C)   Beneficial bacteria found in dairy products
   (D)   A combination of beneficial microbes and carbohydrates

4. Which of the following is an effective pre-exercise warm-up for athletes with EIB

   (A)   High-intensity intermittent exercise
   (B)   Continuous exercise at a low exercise intensity
   (C)   Intermittent resistance exercise
   (D)   Low intensity intermittent exercise

5. Which of the following statements is true?

   (A)   Caffeine supplementation is on the WADA banned list
   (B)   A single espresso shot always contains 6mg of caffeine.
   (C)   Caffeine at a dose of ≤ 10 mg·kg^{-1} causes fluid-electrolyte imbalances.
   (D)   Caffeine at 3, 6 and 9 mg·kg^{-1} consumed 1 hour before exercise reduces EIB severity in a dose dependent manner.

Online resources

Educational information on pre- and probiotics: https://isappscience.org
National Institute for Health information on Omega-3 supplements: https://nccih.nih.gov/
health/omega3/introduction.htm
WADA prohibited list: www.wada-ama.org/en/content/what-is-prohibited

Key reading

Dickinson, J., Amirav, I. & Hostrup M. (2018). Nonpharmacologic strategies to manage exercise-induced bronchoconstriction. *Immunology and Allergy Clinics of North America.*, 38(2), 245–258.

Eichenberger, P. A., Scherer, T. A. & Spengler, C. M. (2016). Pre-exercise hyperpnea attenuates exercise-induced bronchoconstriction without affecting performance. *PloS ONE*, 11(11), e0167318.

Gotshall, R. W., Rasmussen, J. J. & Fedorczak, L. J. (2004). Effect of one week versus two weeks of dietary nacl restriction on severity of exercise-induced bronchoconstriction. *Professionalization of Exercise Physiology*, 7(1), 1–7.

Kurti, S. P., Murphy, J. D., Ferguson, C. S., Brown, K. R., Smith, J. R. & Harms, C. A. (2016). Improved lung function following dietary antioxidant supplementation in exercise-induced asthmatics. *Respiratory Physiology & Neurobiology*, 220, 95–101.

Mickleborough, T. D., Gotshall, R. W., Cordain, L. & Lindley, M. (2001). Dietary salt alters pulmonary function during exercise in exercise-induced asthmatics. *Journal of Sports Sciences*, 19(11), 865–873.

Mickleborough, T., Gotshall, R., Kluka, E., Miller, C. & Cordain, L. (2001). Dietary chloride as a possible determinant of the severity of exercise-induced asthma. *European Journal of Applied Physiology*, 85(5), 450–456.

Mickleborough, T. D., Lindley, M. R. & Montgomery, G. S. (2008). Effect of fish oil-derived omega-3 polyunsaturated fatty acid supplementation on exercise-induced bronchoconstriction and immune function in athletes. *The Physician and Sports Medicine*, 36(1), 11–17.

Millqvist, E., Bengtsson, U. & Löwhagen, O. (2000). Combining a β2-agonist with a face mask to prevent exercise-induced bronchoconstriction. *Allergy*, 55(7), 672–675.

Nisar, M., Spence, D. P., West, D., Haycock, J., Jones, Y., Walshaw, M. J., … & Pearson, M. G. (1992). A mask to modify inspired air temperature and humidity and its effect on exercise induced asthma. *Thorax*, 47(6), 446–450.

Stickland, M. K., Rowe, B. H., Spooner, C. H., Vandermeer, B. & Dryden, D. M. (2012). Effect of warm-up exercise on exercise-induced bronchoconstriction. *Medicine & Science in Sports & Exercise*, 44(3), 383–391.

Tecklenburg, S. L., Mickleborough, T. D., Fly, A. D., Bai, Y. & Stager, J. M. (2007). Ascorbic acid supplementation attenuates exercise-induced bronchoconstriction in patients with asthma. *Respiratory Medicine*, 101(8), 1770–1778.

Van Haitsma, T. A., Mickleborough, T., Stager, J. M., Koceja, D. M., Lindley, M. R. & Chapman, R. (2010). Comparative effects of caffeine and albuterol on the bronchoconstrictor response to exercise in asthmatic athletes. *International Journal of Sports Medicine*, 31 (4), 231–236.

Weiler, J. M., Brannan, J. D., Randolph, C. C., Hallstrand, T. S., Parsons, J., Silvers, W., … & Greenhawt, M. (2016). Exercise-induced bronchoconstriction update – 2016. *Journal of Allergy and Clinical Immunology*, 138(5), 1292–1295.

Williams, N. C., Hunter, K. A., Shaw, D. E., Jackson, K. G., Sharpe, G. R. & Johnson, M. A. (2017). Comparable reductions in hyperpnoea-induced bronchoconstriction and markers of airway inflammation after supplementation with 6· 2 and 3· 1 g/d of long-chain n-3 PUFA in adults with asthma. *British Journal of Nutrition*, 117(10), 1379–1389.

Williams, N. C., Johnson, M. A., Shaw, D. E., Spendlove, I., Vulevic, J., Sharpe, G. R. & Hunter, K. A. (2016). A prebiotic galactooligosaccharide mixture reduces severity of hyperpnoea-induced bronchoconstriction and markers of airway inflammation. *British Journal of Nutrition*, 116(5), 798–804.

Answers: 1 (C), 2 (B), 3 (B), 4 (A), 5 (D)

8

NASAL PROBLEMS IN THE ATHLETE

Guy Scadding

Overview

This chapter will cover:

- Describe and provide definitions for the key sinonasal issues that may affect an athlete.
- Explain why athletes may be more prone to developing sinonasal problems.
- How to clinically assess and diagnose sinonasal problems.
- Discuss the best tools to assess the impact of nasal problems.
- How to logically approach management and provide top tips for allergy avoidance.

Introduction

Athletes are at risk of suffering from allergic rhinitis and related disorders for several reasons. First, rhinitis is extremely common, affecting about 20–25% of the population of most developed countries, alongside rising prevalence in developing nations. Second, athletes are generally young to early middle aged, the time in life during which allergic rhinitis is most prevalent. Third, certain disciplines, particularly endurance disciplines, pool-based disciplines and cold-weather sports, appear to carry a greater risk of suffering with rhinitis (be that allergic rhinitis or non-allergic rhinitis) than aged-matched members of the general population. This may be due to irritant effects – such as chlorine and cold air – or simply greater time spent being exposed to allergens and modifying factors such as pollutants, as in the case of long-distance runners.

What is rhinitis or rhinosinusitis?

In the general population, rhinitis has significant negative impacts on academic and work performance and impairs sleep; in athletes, this is likely to result in impaired performance. Rhinitis is also a risk factor for asthma and can worsen asthma control. Despite this, rhinitis is often not treated or undertreated in athletes, with reluctance to use the mainstay of treatment (i.e. intranasal corticosteroid therapy).

WHAT IS RHINITIS?

Rhinitis means inflammation of the nasal mucosa.

It is characterised by two or more of:

- nose blockage;
- running;
- itching;
- sneezing.

Allergic rhinitis is caused by IgE antibodies to aeroallergens such as dust mites, pollens, animal dander and mould spores.

Rhinosinusitis describes inflammation of the nasal mucosa and paranasal sinuses. It is characterised by nasal congestion/blockage, nasal discharge, facial pain/pressure and hyposmia/anosmia. Both rhinitis and rhinosinusitis may have significant impacts on daily activities, school/work performance, sleep and overall quality of life. These conditions are commonly encountered in athletes, with certain sports associated with particularly high incidence. They may cause troublesome symptoms and reduce quality of life, just as in the general population, and might also impair performance. Treatment is usually straightforward but requires recognition of the problem. Treatment in athletes should follow well-established, evidence-based guidelines with a few additional considerations.

How common is rhinitis in the general population?

Most epidemiological studies have focused on the presence of allergic rhinitis, rather than non-allergic rhinitis. The UK prevalence of allergic rhinitis was estimated at a quarter of adults in a study combining a questionnaire and clinical assessment, including analysis of allergen-sensitisation. Rates in other Westernised populations appear similar. The prevalence ratio of allergic to non-allergic rhinitis is likely to be in the region of 3:1. Both conditions appear to be risk factors for asthma development. The prevalence of doctor-diagnosed chronic rhinosinusitis (CRS) in Europe is 2–4%.

How common is rhinitis in athletes?

Rhinitis is more common in elite swimmers than the general population, with rates reported of between 40 and 74%, and also in cross-country skiers, although a figure of 46% is based on a single study. No such consistent increase was found in other land-based athletes, though sprint/power-based sports seem to be associated with lower prevalence than endurance events. The increased incidence of rhinitis in elite level swimmers may be due to cases of non-allergic rather than allergic rhinitis.

What causes rhinitis?

About three-quarters of rhinitis cases are allergic; that is, mediated by allergen-specific IgE antibodies. The term non-allergic rhinitis describes rhinitis symptoms which occur in the absence of evidence of relevant IgE antibodies as detected by either serum IgE testing or skin prick testing.

Allergic rhinitis may be caused by seasonal and/or perennial allergen exposure and occasionally by allergens encountered at work. In the UK, common seasonal allergens include grass and tree pollens (i.e. wind-dispersed pollens), with house dust mite and cat dander the most important perennial allergens. Mould spores (*Alternaria* spp., *Cladosporium* spp.) may cause problems in late summer and autumn. In North America, ragweed pollen is an important seasonal allergen, as is cedar tree pollen in Japan and *Parietaria* (wall pellitory) pollen in Italy and other parts of Southern Europe. Cockroach allergens are problematic in areas where cockroaches are endemic and often associated with poor quality housing.

Common occupational allergens include flour in bakers and laboratory animal allergens in lab workers. Non-allergic rhinitis may be the result of irritant exposure, medication use and hormone changes (for example, during pregnancy) among other causes.

Acute rhinosinusitis is most frequently the result of viral infection, predominantly rhinovirus (i.e. the common cold virus). Chronic rhinosinusitis, where symptoms last longer than 12 weeks, is generally divided into cases with (CRSwNP) and without nasal polyps (CRSsNP).

The development of allergic sensitisation (i.e. the presence of allergen-specific IgE) requires sufficient allergen exposure, though the relationship between exposure level and sensitisation risk is complex rather than simply linear. A genetic predisposition to atopy (the tendency to produce IgE against allergens) is clearly important, but identification of specific susceptibility genes has proved difficult. Epidemiological evidence suggests factors such as smaller family size, indoor and urban environments, and reduced exposure to infectious disease may be relevant when considering the increased rates of allergic rhinitis seen since the latter part of the twentieth century.

What is the pathophysiology of rhinitis?

In a sensitised individual, upon sufficient allergen exposure at the nasal mucosa, allergen molecules bind and cross-link allergen-specific IgE bound to the surface of mucosal mast cells (Figure 8.1). Sufficient cross-linking results in signal transduction via the high-affinity IgE receptor FcεR1 which leads to mast cell activation and release of secretory granules. These granules contain a number of preformed mediators, such as histamine which stimulates sensory nerve endings within seconds, causing itch and sneezing, dilatation of local vasculature and glandular secretion, leading to nasal blockage and rhinorrhoea. Prostaglandin D2 (PGD2), also released from mast cell granules, is a vasodilator and also promotes influx of T-cells, eosinophils, and basophils. Concurrently, allergen is also taken up by antigen-presenting cells, such as dendritic cells, and presented to T cells. These T-helper 2 type cells secrete interleukins 4 and 13, which stimulate further IgE production from B cells and increased mucous secretion, plus interleukin 5 which stimulates eosinophil recruitment and activation (Figure 8.1). Eosinophils contribute to mucosal damage and inflammation through the release of highly cationic and basic proteins from intracellular granules including ECP (eosinophil cationic protein).

The pathophysiology of non-allergic rhinitis is less well understood and likely differs according to whether or not there is evidence of eosinophilic inflammation. In the absence of eosinophilic inflammation, symptoms are thought to be due to dysfunction of the autonomic nerve supply to the nasal mucosa (excess parasympathetic input, causing gland hypersecretion and capacitance vessel vasodilatation) and/or increased neuropeptide-mediated responses. A typical trigger in these patients is cold, dry air – this may be particularly relevant in skiers and other outdoor winter-based athletes (i.e. causing the typical nasal discharge reported by athletes partaking in these types of sport).

The pathophysiology of rhinitis in elite swimmers may include a non-allergic component. By-products of pool water chlorination include strong anti-oxidants which cause inflammation at the nasal epithelium, including disruption of epithelial tight-junctions. This may allow migration of inflammatory cells across the luminal surface into the nasal cavity with allergens and irritants passing in the opposite direction. Non-allergic rhinitis with eosinophilia (NARES) describes rhinitis with evidence of eosinophilic inflammation (the presence of eosinophils in nasal mucous cytology smears or in histology of nasal turbinate biopsies) without evidence of allergen-specific IgE.

The pathophysiology of chronic rhinosinusitis with nasal polyps (CRSwNP) shares similarities with allergic rhinitis, although the eosinophilic inflammation is usually even more pronounced. The role of IgE in CRSwNP is unclear. The disease may occur in both classically atopic and non-atopic individuals, suggesting allergen-specific IgE is not a prerequisite. Chronic rhinosinusitis without nasal polyps (CRSsNP) probably represents a varied group of pathologies with defects in one or more of mucociliary function, anti-microbial immunity and sino-nasal anatomy.

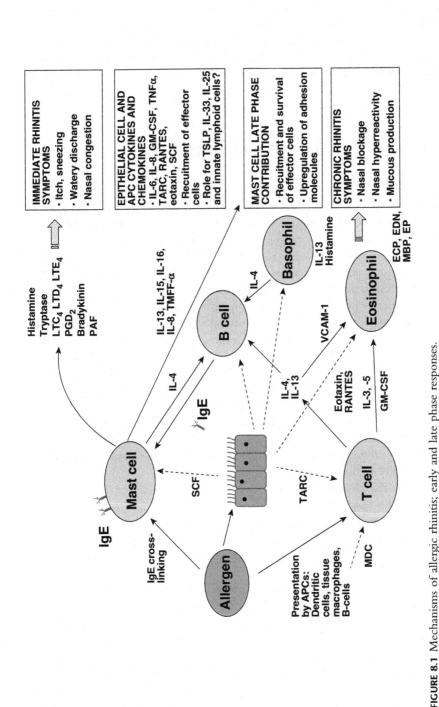

FIGURE 8.1 Mechanisms of allergic rhinitis; early and late phase responses.

ECP, eosinophil cationic protein; EDN, eosinophil-derived neurotoxin; MBP, major basic protein; EP, eosinophil peroxidase; SCF, stem cell factor; MDC, macrophage-derived chemokine.

Source: adapted from Scadding (2008)

The intense exercise necessitated by elite level athletic training may have pathological effects at the nasal mucosa. Swimmers and/or distance runners have been found to have evidence of reduced mucociliary transport time and ciliary beat frequency, reduced phagocytic activity, and increased neutrophils in nasal fluid lavage. Such changes theoretically could increase the risk of upper respiratory tract infection, another frequent problem in elite athletes. Notably, rhinitis symptoms are worse during periods of intense training in elite swimmers, but improve after two weeks away from the pool.

How do I assess an athlete with nasal symptoms?

Take a good history

Rhinitis is defined clinically by the presence of two or more of nasal blockage, running/discharge, itching and sneezing for more than an hour per day. Allergic rhinitis may also present with conjunctivitis in at least 50% of cases. Sneezing, itching and a watery anterior discharge may be particularly predominant in seasonal allergic rhinitis (e.g. hay fever due to grass or tree pollens) and in acute rhinitis prompted by short term exposure to pet allergens.

More chronic exposure, such as perennial exposure to house dust mite allergens or pet allergens within the patient's home, may result in predominant nasal blockage. In children, chronic rhinitis may also present with cough and be misdiagnosed as asthma. Perennial rhinitis in children may also be associated with chronic otitis media with effusion and adenoidal hypertrophy – such features are rarely seen in adults. Individuals with rhinitis may notice symptoms due to non-specific triggers such as cold weather; this reflects the nasal hyperreactivity thought to be due to chronic mucosal inflammation. Patients with allergic rhinitis are also more likely to have or have had other atopic diseases including eczema, asthma and food allergy and/or have a family history of the same.

Non-allergic rhinitis typically presents with either predominant nasal blockage or rhinorrhoea, with less in the way of sneezing and itching (although cases of predominant sneezing and itch may also occur). Hyper-reactivity to non-specific triggers, particularly cold, dry air is well-recognised. Both allergic and non-allergic rhinitis are associated with an increased risk of developing asthma, so lower airway symptoms should be enquired about.

The cardinal features of chronic rhinosinusitis (CRS) are nasal congestion and discharge, particularly a thick, post nasal discharge, with or without facial pressure/pain and reduced or absent sense of smell (the definition according to European consensus guidelines is outlined in the box below). Hyposmia/anosmia is very typical of chronic rhinosinusitis with nasal polyps. Aspirin/NSAID hypersensitivity is also particularly associated with the combination of chronic rhinosinusitis with nasal polyps and asthma.

DEFINITION OF CHRONIC RHINOSINUSITIS (CRS)

Two or more symptoms, one of which should be:

- nasal blockage/congestion or nasal discharge (anterior or post nasal drip); and/or
- facial pain/pressure; and/or
- reduction or loss of smell

... accompanied by:

- endoscopic signs of nasal polyps; and/or
- mucopurulent discharge primarily from middle meatus and/or oedema/ mucosal obstruction primarily in middle meatus; and/or
- mucosal changes within the ostiomeatal complex and/or sinuses on CT

... for ≥12 weeks symptoms without complete resolution of symptoms.

Key examination findings

Signs of allergic rhinitis include mouth breathing, nasal speech, sniffing, nose rubbing (referred to as 'the allergic salute') and throat clearing. A transverse nasal crease may be visible, as well as 'allergic shiners' – dark circles under the eyes, which may be accompanied by so-called Dennie-Morgan folds in the skin beneath the eyes. Patients may have signs of other allergic diseases such as skin changes of eczema and wheeze and cough due to asthma.

The nasal mucosa, viewed either by anterior rhinoscopy (using a head mounted lamp and nasal speculum, or simply an otoscope with the largest attachment) or, ideally, by nasendoscope, is typically swollen, watery and pale (Figure 8.3). Examination of the nasal mucosa in chronic rhinosinusitis should reveal either the presence of nasal polyps in CRSwNP (Figure 8.4) – pale, grey, grape-like structures, usually arising from the middle meatus (the area lateral to the middle turbinate) – or a mucopurulent discharge from the middle meatus and/or oedema in the case of CRSsNP.

What investigations might help?

Skin tests or serum specific IgE tests (previously referred to as RAST tests, but now superseded by ImmunoCAP and other techniques) are required to confirm the presence of allergy, but these should not delay treatment. Skin tests to aeroallergens are safe and inexpensive. Performed on the volar surface of the forearm, they give immediate (15 minute) results and are a useful demonstration to the patient of their sensitisation(s). Conversely, rarer allergens may require serum IgE

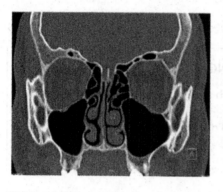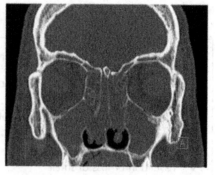

FIGURE 8.2 CT appearances of clear and opacified (chronic rhinosinusitis with nasal polyps) nasal sinuses. With permission.

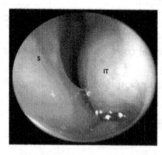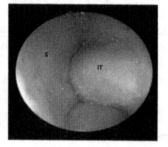

S, nasal septum; IT, inferior turbinate.

FIGURE 8.3 Moderate, left, and severe, right, rhinitis of the anterior nasal mucosa on endoscopic examination. With permission.

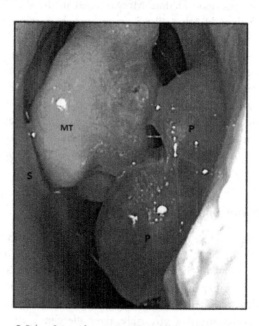

P, Polyp; S, nasal septum; MT, middle turbinate.

FIGURE 8.4 Endoscopic view of the left nasal passage showing nasal polyps. With permission.

tests and skin testing may not be possible in patients with bad eczema or other skin conditions or in those taking anti-histamines. Additional tests may be required depending on the presentation.

Nasal airflow (an indicator of degree of nasal obstruction) can be measured simply using a peak nasal inspiratory flow meter (assuming the patient has normal respiratory muscle function and sniff strength) and is useful in monitoring changes over time/response to treatment. If lower airway symptoms are present then peak flow and spirometry should be considered. In cases of non-allergic rhinitis and CRS a full blood count is helpful for an eosinophil level – higher counts may suggest a more inflammatory, steroid-sensitive process. Additionally, nasal mucous can be sent for cytology to look for eosinophils.

Sinus CT scans may be useful in the diagnosis of CRS, but if the diagnosis is clear from anterior rhinoscopy/nasal endoscopy they should be reserved for patients not responding to medical treatment in whom surgery is to be considered.

How can I assess the impact of rhinitis on athlete health and performance?

Disease-specific quality of life questionnaires for rhinitis are well-validated. The most commonly used is the Rhinitis Quality of Life Questionnaire (RQLQ) or the shorter mini-RQLQ. The disease burden is higher than many healthcare professionals appreciate, with adverse effects on outdoor activities, as well as work and sleep. Academic performance may be impaired in children with grass pollen induced seasonal allergic rhinitis. Concentration and motor skills may also be impaired. Chronic rhinosinusitis disease-specific questionnaires include the SNOT-22.

Concerning athletes, an observational, case-control study found a higher rate of rhinitis in elite swimmers than non-elite swimmers, other athletes and control individuals. This group also had the highest mini-RQLQ scores, indicating the greatest adverse impact on quality of life. Notably, elite swimmers were the least likely group to regularly use medication for their rhinitis. There is some evidence that treatment of rhinitis along standard lines (an intranasal corticosteroid) can lead to an improvement in quality of life scores specifically in elite athletes.

Whether rhinitis and rhinosinusitis have a negative impact on performance in elite athletes remains unproven, but one may speculate that they are likely to do so. Rhinitis may reduce performance on the grounds that it impairs sleep quality. Whether the inflammation or altered nasal airflow dynamics seen in rhinitis and rhinosinusitis have a real-time negative impact on performance is unclear. Finally, again it is worth noting that both rhinitis and chronic rhinosinusitis are strongly associated with asthma which certainly has the potential to reduce exercise performance.

What is the best way to approach to management of nasal symptoms in athletes?

Allergic rhinitis

Identification of allergic triggers on skin prick or serum IgE testing can provide useful information on causative factors. Allergen avoidance in some circumstances can be extremely effective – for example, in cases of occupational rhinitis, removal of or from the trigger can result in complete resolution of symptoms. However, achieving clear benefit in other contexts is often difficult. The exposure burden to perennial allergens such as house dust mite allergen can be reduced by measures including use of allergen proof bedding, reductions in ambient temperature, and removal of carpets and soft furnishings, but such alterations are by no means guaranteed to have a significant impact on symptoms. Avoiding pet allergens should be more straightforward, but animal allergens may remain detectable in the home for months after an animal has left, and in practice people are often very unwilling to turn out a much-loved pet.

Seasonal, outdoor allergens can be avoided by foreign travel, but this is impractical and expensive. Air filtration systems by the bedside have shown positive results, as have nasal filters, albeit only in small trials. With regards to athletes, major championships may cause problems depending on the time of year they are scheduled. Spring and early summer are perhaps the worst times given the high levels of tree and grass pollens. Avoidance of airway irritants, such as cigarette smoke and diesel pollution is also advisable. Simple nasal douching with saline or saline-bicarbonate can be very beneficial both for removal of residual allergen and clearance of excess mucous.

ALLERGEN AVOIDANCE IN ATHLETES – TOP TIPS

Best practised with knowledge of precise sensitisations (by skin testing or serum IgE testing) but clear symptoms on allergen exposure (e.g. typical hay fever in May and June is almost certainly due to grass pollen allergy) is sufficient to consider undertaking allergen avoidance measures:

- For perennial allergens – animal danders, house dust mite – reduction in exposure in the home, particularly the bedroom, is advised. Re-housing of pets may be beneficial; dust mite avoidance measures (hot wash bedding at 60°C, mite-proof bedding, steam-cleaning or removing soft furnishings, reducing humidity) may also help.
- For seasonal allergens – pollens, mould spores – avoid outdoor training in early morning and early evening when pollen levels are at their highest. Shower and wash hair after outdoor exercise.
- Best undertaken alongside use of optimal pharmacotherapy – complete allergen avoidance, aside from training overseas (absence of relevant pollens) or at altitude/areas of low humidity (house dust mite generally live in temperate, humid climates, and not above 1500 metres), is difficult to achieve.

What are the best medications to try to treat rhinitis?

A number of useful guidelines exist concerning the pharmacological management of allergic rhinitis. The ARIA (Allergic Rhinitis and its Impact on Asthma) document provides a simple system for classification and treatment; the BSACI (British Society of Allergy and Clinical Immunology) has recently published updated detailed guidelines and associated algorithm. In brief, mild symptoms can be treated with an as-required non-sedating anti-histamine, but anything more persistent or troublesome should be treated with an intranasal corticosteroid (see Table 8.1). Nasal corticosteroids are more effective than anti-histamines and the combination of anti-histamine and anti-leukotriene (e.g. montelukast). Many preparations are available, but newer drugs with lower systemic bioavailability (mometasone furoate, fluticasone propionate, fluticasone furoate) are preferable. Regular use and correct application are essential for optimal benefit (Figure 8.5). Failure to respond to an intranasal steroid alone should prompt consideration of a combined corticosteroid plus topical anti-histamine preparation. Anti-cholinergic sprays (ipratropium bromide) can help reduce watery rhinorrhoea. Intranasal steroids also have a beneficial effect on allergic conjunctivitis, but more troublesome symptoms warrant treatment with topical sodium cromoglicate, nedocromil sodium or topical antihistamine (azelastine, olopatadine). Athletes should be treated along the same lines.

Oral decongestants should be avoided as elevated urinary levels may be prohibited at competition; oral or intramuscular corticosteroid use may also require a certificate of exemption. (Intramuscular/depot corticosteroid injections are not recommended in the treatment of rhinitis in any guidelines due to risks of adrenal suppression, impaired bone density and necrosis of the femoral head; short courses of oral prednisolone, 15–20 mg daily for up to 7 days, may be used during peak seasonal allergen exposure if all other treatments are proving insufficiently effective). An approach to management of rhinitis is outlined in Figure 8.6.

What is the place of allergen immunotherapy? Should an athlete be desensitised?

This is the practice of repeatedly administering allergen extract to a patient in order to induce clinical and immunological tolerance against the allergen. It involves an alteration in the immune response to the allergen, with a reduction in the allergic Th2 response and an increase in allergen-specific IgG antibodies. In the right patients it can be an extremely effective treatment and have a lasting benefit even after treatment discontinuation. It may be applied by subcutaneous injection or sublingual tablets/drops. Immunotherapy should only be considered in patients where IgE-sensitisation has been demonstrated to the relevant symptom-inducing allergen(s), and usually only for 1 or 2 allergens. It should only be considered in patients who have failed to respond to maximal pharmacotherapy. Treatment, particularly subcutaneous, carries the risk of

TABLE 8.1 Pharmacotherapy for rhinitis and chronic rhinosinusitis

Medication	Indication	Side effects	WADA regulations	Comments
Intranasal corticosteroids	AR, NAR, CRS	Nose bleeding, discomfort	Permitted	Mainstay of treatment; low bioavailability options preferred: FF, FP, MF – safe for long-term use
Intranasal corticosteroid + intranasal antihistamine	AR	As above, plus bitter taste	Permitted?	Evidence of additional benefit over nasal steroid alone – use if insufficient response to nasal steroid
Oral antihistamine	AR	First generation: sedation, antimuscarinic effects	Permitted	Beneficial for itch and sneezing only; avoid first generation; cetirizine good first line choice
Anti-leukotrienes	AR	Nightmares/vivid dreams (rare)	Permitted	Modest effect only
Mast cell stabilisers – e.g. sodium cromoglicate	ARC	Well tolerated	Permitted	Generally only available as eye drops for allergic conjunctivitis
Dual mast cell stabiliser/antihistamine	ARC	Well tolerated	Permitted	As eye drops for allergic conjunctivitis, e.g. olapatadine, ketotifen
Oral corticosteroids	AR, CRS	Acute: insomnia, increased appetite, mood change	Therapeutic exemption required	Effective in AR and CRS with nasal polyps in particular; long-term treatment inadvisable
Decongestants (nasal, oral)	AR, NAR, CRS	Cardiovascular effects if taken orally	Variable, exemption may be required	Effective for nasal obstruction in short term; long term use can worsen congestion
Allergen immunotherapy	AR	Local and systemic reactions, including anaphylaxis	Permitted	Available for a limited number of allergens, only in presence of relevant IgE sensitisation

(Continued)

Table 8.1 (Cont.)

Medication	Indication	Side effects	WADA regulations	Comments
Antibiotics	CRS	Variable; bacterial resistance; gut flora disruption	Permitted	Some evidence for efficacy of 3–12 week courses of antibiotics including azithromycin, clarithromycin, doxycycline

Source: adapted from Steelant et al. (2018)

AR, allergic rhinitis; NAR, non-allergic rhinitis; CRS, chronic rhinosinusitis; FF, fluticasone furoate; FP, fluticasone propionate; MF, mometasone furoate.

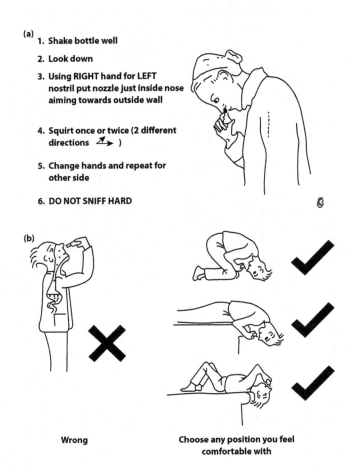

(a)
1. Shake bottle well
2. Look down
3. Using RIGHT hand for LEFT nostril put nozzle just inside nose aiming towards outside wall
4. Squirt once or twice (2 different directions)
5. Change hands and repeat for other side
6. DO NOT SNIFF HARD

(b)

Wrong

Choose any position you feel comfortable with

FIGURE 8.5 How to apply (a) nasal spray and (b) nasal drops.
Source: Scadding, GK et al. 2008

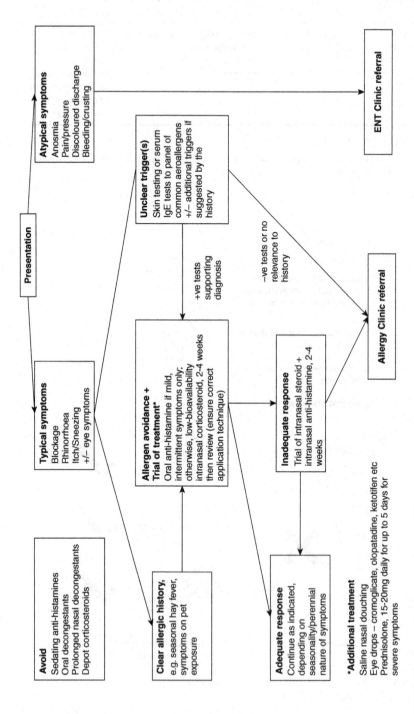

FIGURE 8.6 Approach to management of rhinitis.

Presentation

Typical symptoms
Blockage
Rhinorrhoea
Itch/Sneezing
+/– eye symptoms

Atypical symptoms
Anosmia
Pain/pressure
Discoloured discharge
Bleeding/crusting

ENT Clinic referral

Clear allergic history,
e.g. seasonal hay fever, symptoms on pet exposure

Unclear trigger(s)
Skin testing or serum IgE tests to panel of common aeroallergens +/– additional triggers if suggested by the history

**Allergen avoidance +
Trial of treatment***
Oral anti-histamine if mild, intermittent symptoms only; otherwise, low-bioavailability intranasal corticosteroid, 2-4 weeks then review (ensure correct application technique)

+ve tests supporting diagnosis

–ve tests or no relevance to history

Inadequate response
Trial of intranasal steroid + intranasal anti-histamine, 2-4 weeks

Adequate response
Continue as indicated, depending on seasonality/perennial nature of symptoms

Allergy Clinic referral

Avoid
Sedating anti-histamines
Oral decongestants
Prolonged nasal decongestants
Depot corticosteroids

***Additional treatment**
Saline nasal douching
Eye drops – cromoglicate, olopatadine, ketotifen etc
Prednisolone, 15-20mg daily for up to 5 days for severe symptoms

inducing systemic reactions, including anaphylaxis, and should only be carried out under expert supervision. Poorly controlled asthma is a contraindication.

How should you treat non-allergic rhinitis?

Treatment for non-allergic rhinitis is less evidence based than for allergic rhinitis. First line treatment usually remains an intranasal corticosteroid. In the presence of eosinophilic inflammation (e.g. greater than 5–10% eosinophilia on nasal mucous smear cytology) corticosteroids are more likely to be effective. Other treatment options include nasal ipratropium bromide for those with predominant rhinorrhoea and saline/saline-bicarbonate nasal douching for those with predominant obstruction. In patients with demonstrable nasal hyperreactivity, some centres have had success with use of intranasal capsaicin.

How should you treat chronic rhinosinusitis?

In CRSwNP there is evidence for efficacy of both intranasal and systemic (oral) corticosteroids, though clearly use of the latter in the longer term involves the risk of steroid-induced side effects (in practice low to medium dose oral prednisolone, 5–10mg daily, is only used in patients in whom symptoms are severe despite topical treatments. It is worth noting that such patients often have severe eosinophilic asthma, and oral steroid doses in such patients may be determined more by the asthma than the CRS). Some studies have demonstrated a beneficial effect of longer term courses of oral antibiotics – 8–12 weeks of a macrolide antibiotic, 3–6 weeks of doxycycline – but the evidence for benefit is not overwhelming. Anecdotally, montelukast and other anti-leukotriene drugs may be beneficial in some patients, particularly those with asthma and aspirin-hypersensitivity. Similarly, these patients may be candidates for therapeutic aspirin-desensitisation. Nasal saline irrigation may be beneficial, particularly in post-surgical patients. Surgery (functional endoscopic sinus surgery) is indicated in patients with troublesome symptoms despite the above measures. A number of patients will require repeat surgery in due course; long term use of topical corticosteroids is generally required. New steroid-sparing treatments for severe disease may include both anti-IgE (omalizumab) and anti-IL-5 (mepolizumab), but further large scale trials are required.

In CRSsNP evidence supports the use of intranasal corticosteroids, nasal saline irrigations and, to some extent, extended courses (8–12 weeks) of antibiotics, with most studies performed using macrolides (Fokkens et al. 2012). Failure to respond adequately to medical management should prompt CT scanning of the sinuses and consultation with an ENT surgeon for consideration of sinus surgery. Surgery is aimed at clearing inflammatory material and improving sinus drainage – continuation of medical treatment, principally intranasal steroids and saline irrigations, is generally required in the longer term. Consideration of underlying causes such as antibody deficiency and ciliary dyskinesia should be made, although most cases do not have an apparent predisposing cause. Very asymmetrical disease may indicate a structural abnormality or infection ceded from a dental problem in the case of unilateral maxillary sinusitis.

What is the overall point of treating athletes with nasal symptoms?

Specific evidence of treatment efficacy in elite athletes and subsequent positive impact on performance is very limited, but there is no reason to think that efficacy should be significantly different form the general population. In Olympic and Paralympic athletes with seasonal allergic rhinitis, treatment for 8 weeks with intranasal budesonide resulted in improved symptoms, quality of life and performance scores. Limitations of the referenced study include the open-label format, the subjective questionnaire scoring systems and the 54% return rate of questionnaires. Nonetheless, treatment is to be encouraged, particularly given the apparently low rates of medication use in some elite athletes with rhinitis.

CASE STUDY

Mark is a 23-year-old middle-distance runner. He reports having had hay fever in the summer months since his early teens. In the last 3 years his symptoms have begun earlier in the year, from about March onwards. He takes a daily anti-histamine, but despite this he has nasal and palate itching, itchy, watery eyes, sneezing bouts and a blocked nose; after bouts of sneezing his nose runs profusely. In June he developed a cough and woke in the night with wheeze and difficulty breathing several times. His GP treated him with 5 days of prednisolone tablets.

He attends clinic in July. Examination reveals mouth breathing, nasal speech, occasional nose rubbing and red watery eyes. Examination of the nasal mucosa by endoscopy reveals a pale, watery, swollen mucosa. The chest is clear to auscultation, but his spirometry is mildly obstructive at 4.0/6.0 (ratio 67%, FEV1 85% predicted), with improvement to 4.5/6.1 post salbutamol. Skin prick tests show sensitisation to grass pollens and mixed tree pollens (alder, ash and silver birch), tests to house dust mite, animal danders and moulds are negative.

He is diagnosed with seasonal allergic rhinitis due to tree and grass pollen allergy and allergen-induced asthma. Treatment with intranasal fluticasone propionate spray 100 mcg to each nostril once daily from late February until the end of July the following year is recommended. He is given both inhaled beclomethasone 200 mcg twice daily and inhaled salbutamol 100 mcg 2 puffs as required and instructed to begin regular treatment in February, with the option of reducing to 100mcg inhaled beclomethasone twice daily if free of lower respiratory tract symptoms over the coming months. He will use over the counter sodium cromoglicate eye drops as required, if these are not helpful he needs to be prescribed azelastine or olopatidine eye drops. Should he remain troubled on the above, options include switching to a combined fluticasone-azelastine nasal spray and/or a brief course of oral prednisolone, 20 mg daily for up to 5 days. If he still reports having had troublesome symptoms when he returns to clinic the following summer allergen immunotherapy may be considered.

Conclusion

Nasal congestion and discomfort are very common in the athletic population. Indeed, about a quarter of the population in Westernised countries suffers with allergic rhinitis to some degree, with peak incidence in the third and fourth decades. Additionally, athletes partaking in certain sporting disciplines appear to have a greater than background risk of rhinitis, with elite level swimming seeming to carry the greatest risk. This increased risk may, to a large extent, be the result of an increased incidence of non-allergic (i.e. non IgE-mediated) rhinitis, potentially linked to chlorination in pools. Rhinosinusitis is an important differential diagnosis of rhinitis and differentiating between the two is necessary due to differences in management, particularly the possible need for sinus surgery in chronic rhinosinusitis. Both conditions can significantly impair quality of life and both may both be associated with asthma. Treating these conditions can have a significant impact on symptoms and quality of life and might have benefits for performance in elite athletes.

Summary

- Rhinitis is a problem in about a quarter of the population, particularly young adults; symptoms include two or more of nasal blockage, running, sneezing and itching.
- About 75% of cases are allergic (i.e. IgE-mediated), meaning a quarter of cases are non-allergic; an allergic component can be confirmed by skin prick testing or testing for allergen-specific IgE in serum.
- Knowledge of allergic sensitisation can inform allergen avoidance measures but pharmacotherapy is also required in most cases.
- The mainstay of treatment – for both allergic and non-allergic rhinitis – is intra-nasal corticosteroids with modern drugs with low systemic bioavailability; allergen immunotherapy is an option in cases of confirmed allergy, to a limited range of allergens, if there is an inadequate response to pharmacotherapy.
- Chronic rhinosinusitis involves the paranasal sinuses as well as the nasal mucosa; symptoms include nasal blockage/congestion, thick mucous discharge, facial pressure and, in some cases, loss of smell; first line treatment is pharmacotherapy with intranasal steroids and saline nasal douching; recalcitrant cases may require surgical intervention.

Multiple-choice questions

1. Typical symptoms of allergic rhinitis include:

    (A) Facial pain
    (B) Sneezing
    (C) Rhinorrhoea
    (D) Nasal blockage

2. Reduced sense of smell is typical of which of the following:

    (A)   Allergic rhinitis
    (B)   Non-allergic rhinitis
    (C)   Chronic rhinosinusitis with nasal polyps
    (D)   Chronic rhinosinusitis without nasal polyps

3. Common triggers for allergic rhinitis include

    (A)   House dust mite
    (B)   Grass pollen
    (C)   Cat dander
    (D)   Gluten

4. Examination findings in allergic rhinitis may include:

    (A)   Transverse nasal crease
    (B)   Nasal polyps
    (C)   'Allergic shiners'
    (D)   Turbinate oedema and hypertrophy

5. The most effective pharmacotherapy for allergic rhinitis is:

    (A)   Oral anti-histamine + oral anti-leukotriene
    (B)   Intranasal corticosteroid + intranasal anti-histamine
    (C)   Intranasal corticosteroid + oral anti-histamine
    (D)   Oral anti-histamine + intranasal anti-histamine

Key reading

Bauchau V, Durham SR. Prevalence and rate of diagnosis of allergic rhinitis in Europe. *Eur Respir J.* 2004;24(5):758–764.

Bonini M, Bachert C, Baena-Cagnani CE, Bedbrook A, Brozek JL, Canonica GWet al. What we should learn from the London Olympics. *Curr Opin Allergy Clin Immunol.* 2013;13(1):1–3.

Bougault V, Turmel J, Boulet LP. Effect of intense swimming training on rhinitis in high-level competitive swimmers. *Clin Exp Allergy.* 2010;40(8):1238–1246.

Bousquet J, Schünemann H, Togias A, et al. Next-generation Allergic Rhinitis and Its Impact on Asthma (ARIA) guidelines for allergic rhinitis based on Grading of Recommendations Assessment, Development and Evaluation (GRADE) and real-world evidence. *J Allergy Clin Immunol.* 2019. doi:10.1016/j.jaci.2019.06.049.

Fokkens W, Hellings P, Segboer C. Capsaicin for rhinitis. *Curr Allergy Asthma Rep.* 2016;16(8):60.

Fokkens WJ, Lund VJ, Mullol J, Bachert C, Alobid I, Baroody Fet al. EPOS2012: European position paper on rhinosinusitis and nasal polyps 2012: a summary for otorhinolaryngologists. *Rhinology.* 2012;50(1):1–12.

Hopkins C, Gillett S, Slack R, Lund VJ, Browne JP. Psychometric validity of the 22-item Sinonasal Outcome Test. *Clin Otolaryngol.* 2009;34(5):447–454.

Juniper EF, Thompson AK, Ferrie PJ, Roberts JN. Validation of the standardized version of the Rhinoconjunctivitis Quality of Life Questionnaire. *J Allergy Clin Immunol.* 1999;104(2 Pt 1):364–369.

Katelaris CH, Carrozzi FM, Burke TV, Byth K. Effects of intranasal budesonide on symptoms, quality of life, and performance in elite athletes with allergic rhinoconjunctivitis. *Clin J Sport Med.* 2002;12(5):296–300.

Scadding GK, Durham SR, Mirakian R, Jones NS, Leech SC, Farooque Set al. BSACI guidelines for the management of allergic and non-allergic rhinitis. *Clin Exp Allergy.* 2008;38:19–42.

Scadding GK, Kariyawasam HH, Scadding G, Mirakian R, Buckley RJ, Dixon Tet al. BSACI guideline for the diagnosis and management of allergic and non-allergic rhinitis (Revised Edition 2017; First edition 2007). *Clin Exp Allergy.* 2017;47: 856–889.

Shaaban R, Zureik M, Soussan D, Neukirch C, Heinrich J, Sunyer Jet al. Rhinitis and onset of asthma: a longitudinal population-based study. *Lancet.* 2008;372(9643):1049–1057.

Shamji MH, Durham SR. Mechanisms of allergen immunotherapy for inhaled allergens and predictive biomarkers. *J Allergy Clin Immunol.* 2017;140(6):1485–1498.

Steelant B, Hox V, Hellings PW, Bullens DM, Seys SF. Exercise and sinonasal disease. *Immunol Allergy Clin North Am.* 2018;38(2):259–269.

Surda P, Walker A, Putala M, Siarnik P. Prevalence of rhinitis in athletes: systematic review. *Int J Otolaryngol.* 2017;8098426.

Surda P, Putala M, Siarnik P, Walker A, Bernic A, Fokkens W. Rhinitis and its impact on quality of life in swimmers. *Allergy.* 2017;00:1–10.

Surda P, Walker A, Limpens J, Fokkens W, Putala M. Nasal changes associated with exercise in athletes: systematic review. *J Laryngol Otol.* 2018;18:1–7.

Wilson JM, Platts-Mills TAE. Home environmental interventions for house dust mite. *J Allergy Clin Immunol Pract.* 2018;6(1):1–7.

Answers

1. B, C and D. All are cardinal features of allergic rhinitis. Facial pain is not a typical feature of allergic rhinitis. Pain/pressure over the paranasal sinuses may be a feature of rhinosinusitis.

2. C. Loss of smell (anosmia) or reduced sense of smell (hyposmia) is a typical symptom of chronic rhinosinusitis with nasal polyps; it is less commonly found in chronic rhinosinusitis without nasal polyps and not a typical feature in allergic rhinitis.

3. A, B, C. Allergic rhinitis is triggered by aeroallergens, including pollens, dust mites, animal danders and mould spores; food allergens are seldom the cause of isolated rhinitis symptoms.

4. A, C, D. Transverse nasal crease may be seen, particularly in adolescents, and due to frequent rubbing of the underside of the nose upwards; 'Allergic shiners' refers to the dark circles seen around the eyes, particularly in patients with perennial allergic rhinitis; swelling, pallor and a watery discharge are features of the nasal mucosa (including the turbinates) in allergic rhinitis; nasal polyps are not a feature of allergic rhinitis – their presence is almost invariably associated with sinus inflammation, hence the correct label of chronic rhinosinusitis with nasal polyps.

5.   B. Intranasal corticosteroid + intranasal anti-histamine has been shown to be more effective than either treatment alone; intranasal corticosteroids are more effective than the combination of oral anti-histamine and oral anti-leuko-triene; there is no evidence that taking an oral anti-histamine in addition to an intranasal corticosteroid provides any additional benefit over intranasal corticosteroid alone.

9

EXERCISE-INDUCED LARYNGEAL OBSTRUCTION

J. Tod Olin and Emil S. Walsted

Overview

This chapter will cover:

- What is exercise-induced laryngeal obstruction (EILO).
- How common is EILO and epidemiology.
- What is the typical clinical presentation and how can you diagnose EILO.
- The causes of EILO.
- A logical approach to treating EILO.

Introduction

Exercise-induced laryngeal obstruction (EILO) is an important cause of exertional dyspnea in athletic individuals. It is a condition that has only really been recognised since the 1980s. The condition is defined by the presence of upper airway obstruction at a glottic or supraglottic level during exercise in the absence of associated symptoms at rest.

Since the initial description of the condition, there have been small incremental improvements in the medical community's understanding of disease mechanism. Association of EILO with other forms of laryngeal obstruction and challenges in standardised diagnostic testing initially limited scientific and clinical progress. More recently, clear definitions of the condition and improved diagnostic testing at specialised centres have opened the door to an exciting era which promises more hope to affected patients.

What is inducible laryngeal obstruction?

Inducible laryngeal obstruction (ILO) is an umbrella term, coined and published in 2015 by a multispecialty group of experts, which describes episodic upper airway obstruction caused by the true vocal folds or tissue associated with the arytenoid cartilages, aryepiglottic folds, or epiglottis.

Triggers for these episodes vary across patients and have been categorised in the literature as exercise-related, irritant-related, or associated with mental health disorders. New terminology was specifically proposed to address perceived confusion in the literature and redundancy in terminology (with terms such as vocal cord dysfunction and paradoxical vocal fold motion) which often varied across medical specialty. Moreover, some terms which were associated with the condition including Munchausen's stridor and psychogenic stridor were perceived as potentially stigmatising and possibly acting as barriers to optimal care for patients. At the current time, exercise induced or E-ILO is known as a subgroup of ILO for the purposes of categorisation. Its categorisation as such is not intended to imply mechanistic relationship, but rather to enhance communication among providers of different medical specialties.

What is the impact of EILO?

The impact of EILO on society is challenging to definitively quantitate. Unlike conditions such as asthma or cardiovascular disease, EILO does not lead to tangible mortality or hospital admissions. Rather, its effect is more subtle. First, it is important because it may act as a deterrent to exercise. Quantifying decrements in exercise intensity and quantity, especially among patients that do not present for medical care, is challenging. Secondly, individual patients that present to clinic are often concerned about the effect of the condition on athletic performance. Finally, the literature has described the concept of ILO acting as a mimic of asthma which leads to the consequences of inappropriate therapy with inhaled and oral corticosteroids (as described in the hypothetical case below) and other agents which may lead to unnecessary medication side effects.

How common is EILO?

The prevalence of the condition has been studied. Population prevalence estimates are in the range of 5% in younger populations. However in some studies, the prevalence of EILO has been as high as 20% in athletic individuals undergoing assessment for unexplained exertional breathlessness. There have not been exhaustive studies using rigorous methodologies to estimate prevalence across the age spectrum. These estimates however, despite some limitations of possible ascertainment bias, underscore the fact that EILO is common. Moreover, it will be encountered in a variety of medical settings and for this reason, it is important that both general practitioner and specialist have an understanding of the typical presentation of EILO as well as suggested evaluation and treatment practices. Many series describe a female predominance among affected patients as well as descriptions of perfectionistic personality tendencies.

Why does EILO develop?

The defining features of EILO are upper airway obstruction that occurs during exercise and temporal association of this obstruction with perceptions of exertional dyspnea. The mechanisms through which these occur are not clearly elucidated and may vary across individual patients. It is clear that there is a notable increase in airflow resistance and neural drive in those experiencing current symptoms. Some authors have described similarities between the upper airways of EILO patients and those of patients with congenital laryngomalacia. If there were, indeed, a demonstrated statistical association between the two conditions, it may be reasonable to conclude that airway pliability and absolute airway size contribute to the likelihood of symptoms and/or disease.

There is likely is to be an association between EILO symptoms and other causes of upper airway irritation. If causally linked, these observations may suggest that neural processes may play a role. One can hypothesise within this line of thinking that epithelial barrier function, afferent signalling, efferent signalling, or muscular function may affect the frequency and severity of symptoms. Other potentially relevant factors include gastroesophageal reflux; potentially via its effect as a direct irritant or as a neurologic contributing factor. Post nasal drip has also been hypothesised to contribute.

The role of psychological distress is unclear. Many descriptions of ILO and EILO have included observations about behavioural health features, such that an association between the two seems accepted. At the same time, causal links are unclear. It is possible that some behavioural features may be a result of symptoms rather than a cause.

Understanding of the role of asthma and its overlap with ILO is evolving. It is clear that a proportion of athletes with EILO also have asthma (confirmed with bronchoprovocation testing) and this may confound and complicate the diagnosis and symptom assessment of EILO. Moreover, lower airways disease may notably affect upper airway behaviour through neurophysiologic coupling.

How does EILO present clinically?

Many of the prototypical EILO cases that have been published describe frightening exertional inspiratory stridor which occur almost exclusively during very high-intense exercise. Cough may or may not be present. Symptoms often rapidly resolve upon termination of exercise with duration of symptoms somewhat associated with the peak severity of symptoms. Pallor, presyncope, and syncope can occur and may possibly be linked with dysfunctional respiratory patterns that occur as a secondary phenomenon to upper airway obstruction.

CASE STUDY

A 21-year-old female university athlete who competes in the 400 m and 800 m events presents for a second medical opinion regarding her eight months of exertional stridor. She has no prior history of asthma or allergy. She does not cough and denies pallor, presyncope, cyanosis, and syncope. She describes notable fear which associates with the symptom as well as concern among bystanders for her respiratory symptoms. Symptoms are most prominent during the final 30 seconds of her 800 m run as well as during training sessions which feature high-intensity interval sprint work. Symptoms occur during nearly roughly 75% of high-intensity training sessions and can resolve within 30 seconds of exercise termination. With respect to environmental factors that could affect the frequency and severity of symptoms, she feels most affected at the extremes of ambient temperature. She has not responded symptomatically to salbutamol four puffs 15 minutes prior to exercise. At baseline, she describes frequent throat clearing and a globus sensation as well as congestion and rhinorrhea that are most prominent while present in grassy outdoor environments in the spring.

The medical provider suggests a diagnosis of EILO is highly likely. The patient becomes frustrated because previous evaluations for the condition, including multiple laryngoscopies (at rest, after methacholine, after mannitol, and after exercise) have not clearly identified the presence of EILO.

In reality, our anecdotal experience calls attention to the variability of clinical presentation and some pitfalls in acquisition of the history. Cough, traditionally felt to be suggestive of asthma anecdotally is seen on occasion as an apparently compensatory response to the stridor described above. Stridor is not universally described as the presence or absence of stridor may be a function of obstruction severity and absolute airflow. Characterisation of inspiratory versus expiratory limitation may be misleading for its lack of specificity. While patients with EILO often appropriately characterise inspiratory limitation, it is our experience that many patients with severe expiratory disease including asthma, cystic fibrosis, and chronic obstructive pulmonary disease often inappropriately make the same characterisation (Table 9.1, Figure 9.1).

Physical exam findings at rest are generally normal with respect to specific respiratory findings. Stigmata of allergic disease another sinonasal disease may be present. It is our experience that low intensity exercise observations and basic clinic settings are not sufficient to reproduce exam findings of relevance for EILO.

What are the other causes of EILO-type symptoms?

Among adolescent and young adult populations, asthma must be considered once dyspnea has been clearly identified as it is the most commonly encountered respiratory disease and the majority of patients with asthma experience exertional symptoms (see Chapter 5).

TABLE 9.1 Differences between EILO and EIB

	EILO	*EIB*
Onset	Fast onset 1–5 minutes after starting high intensity exercise	Slow onset 15–30 minutes after starting high intensity exercise
Duration	0–5 minutes after exercise cessation	30–60 minutes or longer after exercise cessation
Location	Throat or upper chest	Chest
Characteristics (not always present)	'Like breathing through a straw' Throat tightness or pain Cough Inspiratory stridor	Chest tightness Cannot get a deep satisfying breath Expiratory wheeze Cough
short-acting β_2-agonist response	No change	Attenuates symptoms

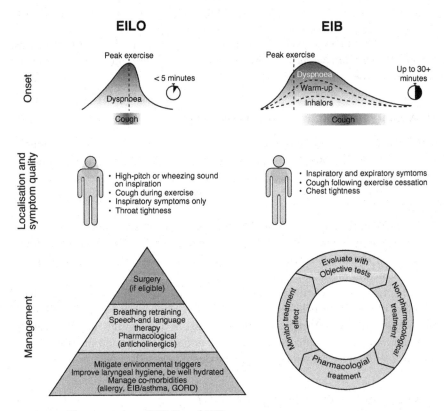

FIGURE 9.1 Characteristics of EILO and EIB.
EIB, exercise-induced bronchoconstriction; EILO, exercise- induced laryngeal obstruction.
Source: adapted from Griffin et al. (2018).

Other forms of pulmonary, cardiac, and pulmonary vascular disease can also certainly present with exertional dyspnea. An exhaustive enumeration of these conditions is beyond the scope of this chapter, but the possibility of these conditions is important when diagnostic testing protocols are considered.

If stridor has been convincingly described, healthcare providers should consider all forms of intrinsic large airway obstruction and extrinsic large airway compression. These lesions may include subglottic stenosis, endobronchial cysts, vascular malformations, and compression from thoracic vasculature or masses. Importantly, these fixed lesions intuitively should not cause symptoms that vary in intensity across exercise bouts of similar intensity.

Breathing pattern disorders (also known as dysfunctional breathlessness) may cause some symptoms which overlap with EILO (see Chapter 11). A key similarity between the two conditions are the ability of both EILO and dysfunctional breathing to act as a mimic to asthma.

A key difference between the two conditions is the presence of symptoms at rest among most patients with dysfunctional breathing.

Another condition which causes visibly noisy breathing almost exclusively during exercise is known as excessive dynamic airway collapse. It is a recently described phenomenon which is characterised by dynamic large airway collapse leading to symptomatic airflow limitation with symptoms almost exclusively isolated to exercise.

How can you make a diagnosis of EILO?

The evaluation of patients with suspected EILO should focus on characterisation of upper airway behaviour during periods of self-identified symptom reproduction. Importantly, an evaluation should also simultaneously include assessment of asthma (a more common diagnosis which can also coexist with EILO) and potential disease contributors.

Providers in a variety of clinical settings can accomplish some of these latter objectives. Spirometry +/− bronchodilator testing (i.e. in the presence of airflow obstruction) can be an initial screen for the presence or absence of reversible airflow obstruction that is seen in asthma (see Chapter 5)

Provocative asthma testing with eucapnic voluntary hyperventilation, inhaled mannitol challenge, or field testing in specific environments is best accomplished in subspecialty practice. Allergy skin prick testing is a relatively simple screen for allergic rhinitis (see Chapter 8). Imaging for sinonasal disease and physiologic testing for gastroesophageal reflux can be considered in specific cases.

How do you specifically test for EILO?

The specific evaluation of EILO has been challenging since the initial description of the disease. A variety of modalities has been used historically in practice and in the literature. These have included assessment through clinical history alone and non-invasive methods including flow volume loop analysis, ultrasonographic assessment, and impulse oscillometry. More invasive approaches have included resting laryngoscopy, post-exercise laryngoscopy, pre-and post-exercise laryngoscopy, post-surrogate challenge laryngoscopy, and continuous laryngoscopy during exercise (CLE). The complexity, fruitfulness, and potential for these procedures to mislead varies importantly.

We strongly and specifically advocate for the use of CLE for the definitive assessment of EILO. This is a procedure which features direct laryngoscopic visualisation continuously during an incremental bout of exercise. It can be performed in association with electrocardiographic, ventilatory, and metabolic data collection, which can be critical in the identification or exclusion of conditions in the differential diagnosis (Figure 9.2). Depending on available resources, the procedure can be performed and has been described during cycle ergometry, treadmill ergometry, rowing, and even swimming (Figure 9.3).

We advocate for the use of CLE, aware of the logistic burdens of the procedure, for multiple reasons. Most importantly, CLE enables upper airway visualisation during intense exercise minimising the possibility of a falsely negative endoscopic evaluation. The time course of visualised upper airway obstruction among patients with EILO has been described in the literature. It is critical to understand that, in the vast majority of patients, upper airway obstruction in patients with EILO is not present at rest, during submaximal exercise, or after the immediate phases of recovery. Additionally, CLE has the potential to minimise falsely positive evaluations as well. Post-exercise laryngoscopy can be uncomfortable, especially if per-

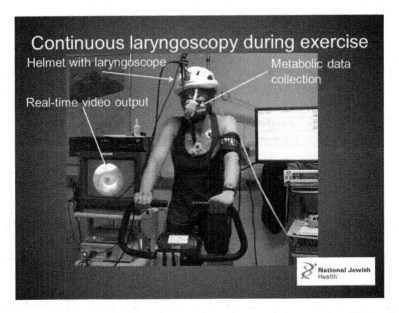

FIGURE 9.2 Equipment set-up for continuous laryngoscopy during exercise (CLE) testing. Source: provided courtesy of T. Olin

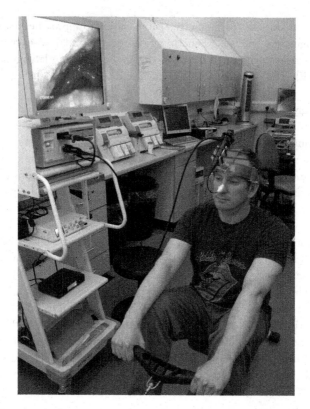

FIGURE 9.3 Continuous laryngoscopy during exercise testing during rowing. Source: provided courtesy of J. Hull

formed by proceduralists without extensive experience in patients experiencing sudden onset shortness of breath. The guarding behaviours and occasional vocalisations induced in patients by the procedure can cause upper airway changes which mimic EILO. While not definitively quantitated in the literature, the teaching value of CLE footage for patients is notable possibly because many young patients express a desire to observe findings during symptomatic periods of time.

We do not advocate for the use of laryngoscopy during or after surrogate challenges. Many of the surrogate challenges (including methacholine, eucapnic voluntary hyperventilation, and mannitol) were specifically designed to evaluate asthma. Some have been definitively shown to not trigger EILO. The biologic possibility that these conditions would also consistently, sensitively, and specifically elicit another disease in addition to asthma seems doubtful. Moreover, it is our anecdotal experience that patients can lose some confidence in the diagnostic process when providers (repeatedly) express concern for false negative evaluations (as described in the case presentation above).

Although the procedure can be performed in the absence of simultaneous exercise data collection and expertise in exercise physiology, we caution centres considering this approach. While cardiac, ventilatory, and metabolic data are not specifically required to make a diagnosis of EILO, they can be informative of other conditions and for monitoring the safety of patients. Overall, an approach to the assessment and diagnosis process is presented in Figure 9.4.

What is the best way to treat EILO?

The literature has documented a variety of therapeutic options for EILO. These can be characterised as medical, surgical, and behavioural. It is important to understand the randomised clinical trials data does not exist to quantitatively assess the relative benefits of these interventions.

The important medical therapies for the condition should address potentially contributing our coexisting diagnoses including asthma, sinonasal disease, and gastroesophageal reflux. We reiterate that these conditions are not definitively proven to cause EILO. Moreover, studies which have treated these conditions in isolation have never been shown to improve EILO symptoms. Nonetheless, these conditions are important in their own right and warrant attention, especially in symptomatic patients.

What are the medical therapy options for EILO?

Specific medical therapy for EILO has been proposed. There are reports of the use of inhaled anticholinergic agents, using a rationale that muscarinic signalling

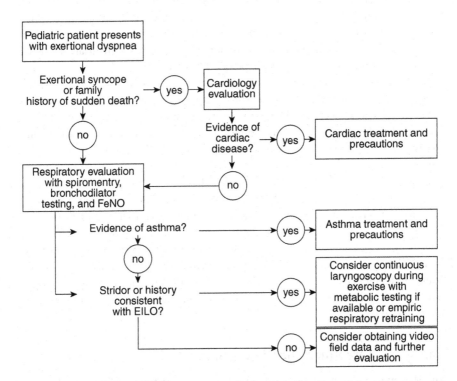

FIGURE 9.4 Diagnostic algorithm in the assessment of unexplained breathlessness and potential EILO.

pathways are central to the inappropriate upper airway behaviour. There are reports of tricyclic antidepressant therapy for patients with ILO. The data behind both of these therapies is weak and subject to many biases such that we cannot definitively recommend use of these agents at this time although the authors do recognise the low risk of harm caused by inhaled anticholinergic agents.

Focal injections of botulinum toxin have also been reported in the literature. This intervention has been reported from a relatively small number of centres. Case series data demonstrates and effectiveness signal that warrant future study of the procedure. As with supraglottoplasty, publication bias may lead to underestimation of procedural complications.

There are a number of behavioural interventions for EILO, and some of these are considered first-line therapies for the condition.

Speech-language pathology intervention may include a number of different features. Motor retraining of upper airway muscles is hypothesised to explain the benefits reported in case series. Specific techniques range from simple to complex. Initial techniques described focused on pursed lip exhalation and attention to diaphragmatic breathing. More recently, a complex manoeuvre called the EILOBI technique was described, its creation based on direct visualisation during performance of the manoeuvre.

Inspiratory muscle training has also been reported as a therapy for EILO. The mechanisms through which this intervention may improve the condition are unclear, although they may be related to changes in perception of dyspnea. Inspiratory muscle training involves the use of an inspiratory resistor as a strengthening device for inspiratory muscles. Resistance can be systematically increased over time to optimise training protocols (see Chapter 12).

Biofeedback, broadly defined, is the real-time use of biologic data to guide responses of an individual. This concept has been described as a potential therapy for EILO. Airflow patterns which graphically quantitate and respiratory rate have been used to improve control of respiration. In recent years, the use of real-time laryngoscopy has been described as a respiratory modulator for patients with EILO.

Finally, behavioural health interventions have been proposed as adjunctive therapy for ILO and EILO. These treatment modalities have been considered with the rationale that there are some common behavioural observations made among groups of patients. While there may be differences between the initial reports of ILO patients struggling with symptoms outside of exercise and patients with isolated EILO, therapy directed at some of the perfectionistic tendencies could be beneficial as a secondary therapy. Additionally, consideration of cognitive-behavioural therapy with a primary focus on the demands of sport warrants future study.

Can surgical treatment be beneficial in EILO?

Surgical approaches have been advocated for the treatment of EILO with predominant supraglottic contribution, mainly by large centres based in Europe. Some of the initial descriptions of surgical intervention cited an observation that patients with supraglottic disease had airway configurations conceptually similar to infants with congenital laryngomalacia. The rationale behind the use of supraglottoplasty in the treatment of EILO is that many patients have surgical changes in airway aperture at a supraglottic level can have fairly profoundly beneficial theoretic impacts on airway resistance. At the current time, we think it is reasonable to consider surgery in select cases of supraglottic EILO, realising that there is a paucity of long-term safety data and the potential for publication bias which could under-estimate procedural complications.

Conclusion

EILO is an important condition because it is common and may act as a deterrent in an age when exercise is promoted as a primary prevention or therapy for a number of medical conditions. Its relatively recent discovery in the 1980s con-tributes to the relative lack of mechanistic knowledge about the condition. It can exist in isolation or in combination with asthma and other conditions. For this reason, it should not be evaluated in isolation. CLE is the preferred diagnostic method to assess EILO although there are challenges to performing and inter-preting the test. Behavioural interventions including speech-language pathology are the first-line therapies for the condition. Surgery can be considered in select cases of predominantly supraglottic disease. Medical therapy cannot be recom-mended at the current time although the relative risk of inhaled anticholinergic agents is low.

Summary

- Exercise-induced laryngeal obstruction (EILO) describes a transient narrowing of the laryngeal inlet that occurs during strenuous exercise. It has also been historically known as vocal cord dysfunction and paradoxical vocal fold motion.
- EILO affects roughly 5% of the adolescent and young adult population and leads to respiratory symptoms which may cause a decrease in performance and willingness to participate in sport.
- The mechanism of EILO is not fully elucidated, and is hypothesised to result from abnormalities in airway anatomy, inflammatory biology, neurologic priming, dysfunctional motor patterns, and possibly psychology.
- EILO clinically presents as exertional dyspnea with rapid onset and short duration, localising to the throat, often in the context of audible inspiratory stridor.
- EILO has been treated medically, surgically, and behaviourally at different centres globally. Respiratory retraining as directed by a speech-language pathologist is the mainstay of therapy currently.

Multiple choice questions

1. What testing modality best detects EILO?

   (A) Pre-/post exercise spirometry
   (B) Post exercise laryngoscopy
   (C) Continuous laryngoscopy during exercise
   (D) Cardiopulmonary exercise test

2. Patient reported symptoms can be used to detect EILO

   (A) Yes, if gathered via structured interviews / questionnaires
   (B) Yes, but only in individuals without concomitant asthma
   (C) No, but symptoms provide useful clinical clues
   (D) No, patient reported symptoms have no place in the investigation of EILO

3. When and individual has both EILO and EIB …

   (A) It may be feasible to step down asthma medication
   (B) Inhaler treatment should likely be stepped up
   (C) It is usually clear which of the conditions contributes the most to symptoms
   (D) ACQ or ACT questionnaires can be used to guide asthma treatment

4. The appropriate first-line treatment strategy for EILO is …

   (A) Inhaled corticosteroids
   (B) Non-invasive non-pharmaceutical interventions
   (C) Supraglottoplasty
   (D) Inhaled anticholinergics

5. EILO is estimated to be present in …

   (A) 5% of elite athletes
   (B) 5% of individuals with asthma
   (C) 5% of the general population
   (D) 5% of the young general population

Key reading

Christensen PM, Heimdal JH, Christopher KL, et al. ERS/ELS/ACCP 2013 International Consensus Conference nomenclature on inducible laryngeal obstructions. *Eur Respir Rev.* 2015;24(137):445–450.

Griffin SA, Walsted ES, Hull JH. Breathless athlete: exercise-induced laryngeal obstruction. *Br J Sports Med.* 2018; 52:1211–1212.

Hall A, Thomas M, Sandhu G, Hull JH. Exercise-induced laryngeal obstruction: a common and overlooked cause of exertional breathlessness. *The British Journal of General Practice: the Journal of the Royal College of General Practitioners.* 2016;66(650):e683–685.

Halvorsen T, Walsted ES, Bucca C, et al. Inducible laryngeal obstruction: an official joint European Respiratory Society and European Laryngological Society statement. *Eur Respir J.* 2017;50(3): 1602221.

Heimdal JH, Roksund OD, Halvorsen T, Skadberg BT, Olofsson J. Continuous laryngo-scopy exercise test: a method for visualizing laryngeal dysfunction during exercise. *Laryngoscope*. 2006;116(1):52–57.

Johansson H, Norlander K, Berglund L, et al. Prevalence of exercise-induced bronchocon-striction and exercise-induced laryngeal obstruction in a general adolescent population. *Thorax*. 2015;70(1):57–63.

Johnston KL, Bradford H, Hodges H, Moore CM, Nauman E, Olin JT. The Olin EILOBI breathing techniques: description and initial case series of novel respiratory retraining strategies for athletes with exercise-induced laryngeal obstruction. *J Voice*. 2017;32 (6):698–704.

Maat RC, Roksund OD, Olofsson J, Halvorsen T, Skadberg BT, Heimdal JH. Surgical treatment of exercise-induced laryngeal dysfunction. *Eur Arch Otorhinolaryngol*. 2007;264 (4):401–407.

Norlander K, Johansson H, Jansson C, Nordvall L, Nordang L. Surgical treatment is effec-tive in severe cases of exercise-induced laryngeal obstruction: A follow-up study. *Acta Otolaryngol*. 2015;135(11):1152–1159.

Olin JT, Clary MS, Fan EM, et al. Continuous laryngoscopy quantitates laryngeal behaviour in exercise and recovery. *Eur Respir J*. 2016;8(4):1192–1200.

Olin JT, Deardorff EH, Fan EM, et al. Therapeutic laryngoscopy during exercise: A novel non-surgical therapy for refractory EILO. *Pediatr Pulmonol*. 2017;52(6):813–819.

Olin JT, Westhoff Carlson E. Exercise-Induced Laryngeal Obstruction and Performance Psychology: Using the Mind as a Diagnostic and Therapeutic Target. *Immunology and Allergy Clinics of North America*. 2018;38(2):303–315.

Answers: 1 (C), 2 (C), 3 (A), 4 (B), 5 (D)

10

DEALING WITH RESPIRATORY INFECTION IN ATHLETES

James H. Hull and Glen Davison

Overview

This chapter will cover:

- The impact and importance of respiratory tract infection in athletic individuals.
- Describe if athletes are truly more susceptible to respiratory tract infection and address the potential reasons why.
- Highlight the key infective pathogens relevant in causing respiratory tract infection in athletes.
- Address how best to assess and treat an athlete presenting with acute upper respiratory tract symptoms, with due consideration for return to play.
- Provide pragmatic strategies to reduce risk of respiratory tract infection in athletes.

Introduction

It is generally accepted that moderate amounts of exercise improve immune system function and hence exercise has the potential to reduce susceptibility to the development of respiratory tract infection (RTi). In contrast, however, it is also believed that athletes engaged in regular prolonged and/or intensive training, particularly in noxious or certain challenging environments, appear to have a higher than 'normal' incidence of RTi.

When RTi develops in a competitive athlete it has immediate implications, with impact on performance capability, either directly (i.e. if suffered shortly before or during competition), or indirectly (i.e. affecting training and/or physiological adaptations). Indeed, acute RTi is the most common reason an elite athlete seeks medical assistance during major competitions, with a high prevalence of RTi consistently demonstrated and reported throughout major international sporting tournaments (e.g. at international swimming competitions and Olympic games).

The reasons an athlete might demonstrate increased susceptibility to RTi are complex and likely arise as an imbalance between factors that weaken or compromise the athlete's host defence mechanisms, but also arise from the interplay with environmental risks and exposure factors. Recognised and reported influences include the deleterious impact of psychological stress, extreme environmental exposure, sleep deprivation, airline travel and relative energy deficiency (Figure 10.1).

In the athlete presenting acutely with upper RTi symptoms, evaluation can be challenging. A clinical-based approach to diagnosis is clearly important but also in many ways suboptimal and diagnostically flawed. Athletes presenting with non-specific respiratory tract symptoms are most often treated with antibiotics, with a fear that not 'covering' a potential bacterial infection may run the risk of a delay in treatment and thus the potential for more serious complications that may include a delay to return to competition/full training. This approach risks a treatment strategy targeting non-existent bacterial infection and indeed exposes athletes to the deleterious effects of some groups of antibiotics (e.g. gastrointestinal side effects, development of tendinopathy).

Overall therefore any practitioner or clinician who is involved in the care of athletes must have a good understanding of the factors that contribute to the development of infection, the relevant potential pathogenic mechanisms and the most logical and pragmatic approach to treatment; bearing in mind considerations for anti-doping regulations and 'return to play'.

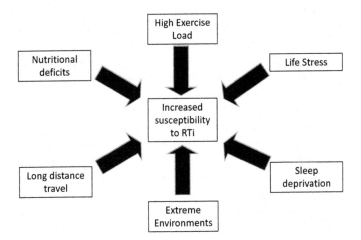

FIGURE 10.1 Key factors impacting immune function in athletic individuals.
Source: adapted from Walsh (2018)

This chapter thus aims to help practitioners faced with this challenge, by providing a pragmatic summary of the key factors when considering symptoms of RTi in athletic individuals. The chapter begins by considering the epidemiology of RTi before considering the pathogenesis and aetiology then focussing on providing a practitioner's approach to assessment and treatment.

HOW DO I KNOW IF AN ATHLETE SHOULD BE CONSIDERED 'SUSCEPTIBLE' TO RTI

It is estimated that in the northern hemisphere, the average person will typically experience between 2 and 3 upper RTi episodes per year. Thus, generally-speaking, if an athlete is having recurrent (i.e. >2 episodes per year) of RTi events that are impacting on training and/or competition (i.e. with an associated loss of training/availability days), it is paramount that a thorough review of their respiratory health and infection susceptibility is undertaken.

Are respiratory tract infections really more common in athletes?

It is a long-standing notion and widely held belief that a 'J-shaped relationship' exists between exercise workload and susceptibility to upper RTi (Figure 10.2, solid lines). i.e. both low and very high levels of regular physical activity are associated with an increased risk of immune system vulnerability and by virtue of this an increased risk of infection. It has been suggested that many athletes will fall to the right-hand side of this curve; i.e. associated with an above-average risk of RTi. This is particularly pertinent in endurance athletes such as cyclists, runners, swimmers, and triathletes, but any athletes with a high training load and/or sub-optimal recovery may be at increased risk.

More recently, it has been proposed that this relationship may actually conform to more of an S-type configuration (Figure 10.2, broken lines), in that super-elite athletes (i.e. those at the very peak of their respective sport) appear to have relatively fewer RTi and thus appear to be 'protected' against infection. This of course may be a prerequisite to them actually achieving this 'elite' athletic status in the first instance; i.e. having an immune system which can withstand the strenuous nature of training and competition to withstand the rigors and challenges mandated by elite training. The reason super-elite athletes appear protected is currently unknown and may relate to genetic advantages in immune function/host defence. It is also however relevant that elite/professional athletes typically have considerable support (financial, medical, sports science and nutrition, etc.), i.e. they are able to implement preventive and treatment strategies to mitigate the risk factors (as mentioned in Figure 10.1), thereby reducing risk and are able to better instigate preventive management strategies and modulate reversible factors.

Regardless of whether or not the most very elite athletes suffer fewer URTI episodes (in total) per calendar year compared to other athletes, there is evidence

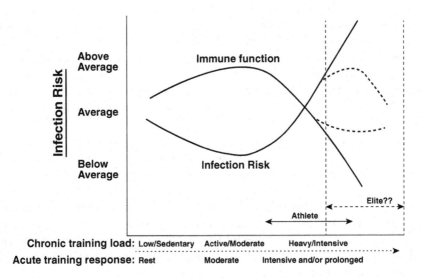

FIGURE 10.2 Relationship between infection risk, physical activity level and training load.

that heavy training is associated with altered immune susceptibility and RTi incidence increases in athletes around intensive periods of training, training camps, and
major competitions that last several days or weeks (e.g. Olympic games or World
Championships events).

What are the factors that may make an athlete more susceptible to infection?

Many components of the immune system are temporarily reduced after strenuous
and/or prolonged bouts of exercise. This exercise-induced immunodepression may
persist for as little as a few hours or a long as a few days, depending on the nature
of the exercise load undertaken. Specifically, if repeated exercise bouts are undertaken too frequently, before the immune system has fully recovered, then a progressive accumulation of immunodepression may ensue. Periods of depressed
immunity, whether for short duration/acute periods or more chronic periods, are
termed 'open windows' (i.e. a time when immune suppression/modulation permits
increased susceptibility). It is important to point out however that this does not
necessarily mean that changes in isolated immune markers alone can predict illness
risk and environmental, exposure and other controllable risk factors (as mentioned
above and in Figure 10.1) are also important.

Is training load relevant in the risk of an athlete developing RTi?

By virtue of their occupation, many elite athletes must train intensively and regularly, meaning they are at an increased risk of RTi for considerable periods of

time (i.e. a greater number or duration of *open window periods*). The relationship between acute and/or chronic exercise is very specific to an induvial athlete (and will vary with training status, training phase etc.), so it is difficult to identify specific exercise intensities, durations and loads associated with increased risk in a given athlete. However, generally speaking, prolonged (>90 min) exercise at ~55–75% maximal aerobic capacity is suggested as a 'tipping point' to increase susceptibility.

High chronic training loads have also been linked to the risk of such illnesses, although some studies suggest those with the highest training loads have ironically been associated with lower risk. Certainly, sudden intensified training periods and training camps appear to be associated with increased risk, although this may relate to 'exposure' risk (i.e. co-habiting with other athletes who may be unwell, and travel).

Overall, it appears that rapid increases in training load/stimulus may be a key risk factor (more so than total training load per se) for RTi occurrence in athletes and taken together, this suggests that it is not simply overall training load, but how this is distributed and periodised that is most important.

What lifestyle and other risk factors may make an athlete susceptible to infection?

Several factors are likely to be relevant in increasing the risk of developing RTi. Factors identified include psychological stress, personal or life stresses, exposure to infected individuals, inadequate diet, lack of sleep and complex travel.

Viral challenge studies (e.g. with the most prevalent cause of the common cold, rhinovirus) in humans have suggested that the likelihood of developing infection is 4-fold greater in those who had <6 h vs > 6 h sleep per night in the week prior to viral challenge. Thus to avoid infection it is generally recommended that athletes should aim for at least 7 hours of high-quality sleep per day and can consider monitoring sleep duration and efficiency with modern wearable devices. Optimising sleep hygiene routines in the few hours prior to bed (e.g. going screen free), can be difficult to practically implement with modern day elite/professional athletes but are likely to be rewarding in terms of enhanced sleep and thus immune function optimisation.

Likewise, it is important not to overlook or discount the importance of either hidden or revealed stressors in modulating immune functions. Several studies have now shown an interplay between heightened psychological stress and immune modulation. Any coach or medical structure will already be cognisant of this aspect of the holistic care of an athlete but in those who appear susceptible to recurrent infection, it is worth re-visiting this component of care.

How can you reduce exposure to infection?

Regardless of immune status or 'host' factors, infection is also dependent on exposure to pathogens. Sometimes this may be beyond an athlete's control, but some strategies can be employed to reduce or minimise exposure; for example giving advice to avoid crowded places, contact with infected individuals, isolate infected team mates from others. It is also vital that athletes have detailed training on optimal hand-washing technique and this is reinforced and repeated on a regular basis. It should be made clear that simply rapidly soaking your hands is not an effective way to reduce infective pathogen exposure (Figure 10.3).

For competitive / elite athletes a key and repeatedly reported risk factor for infection is airline travel. Confined exposure for many hours, in this context, increases the risk of exposure to infection, not only via confined aerosolising of infective pathogens but also via direct contact. Strategies to avoid infection exposure during plane travel include: (i) avoiding sitting next to passengers with obvious features of infection (e.g. sneezing and coughing), and if this is unavoidable then wearing a protective mask; (ii) sitting away from the aisle seats; (iii) consider that risk is greater when travelling west to east; and (iv) remaining well hydrated.

Are athletes travelling or training in extreme training environments at increased risk of infection?

It is apparent that athletic individuals who are exposed to cold, wet and inhospitable (i.e. exposed) environments are more likely to sustain subsequent infection. The following recommendations have thus been suggested to try and maintain immune health in this scenario.

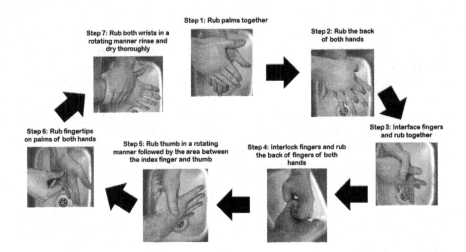

FIGURE 10.3 The seven steps of handwashing.

RECOMMENDATIONS TO MAINTAIN IMMUNE HEALTH IN ATHLETES ENCOUNTERING EXTREME ENVIRONMENTS

1. Carefully manage training load and recovery when training with additional heat and/or hypoxia
2. Acclimation to heat and/or hypoxia may limit the influence of environmental extremes on immune health
3. Take extra precautions to avoid prolonged periods breathing large volumes of cold, dry air e.g. when training and competing in the winter
4. Personal hygiene, sleep hygiene, proper nutrition and reducing unnecessary stress become increasingly important during long-haul travel to training camps and competition
5. Short-lasting exposure to environmental extremes may enhance immunity and reduce sickness e.g. 30s (hot-to)-cold showers

Reproduced from Walsh (2018)

Can dietary modifications be helpful in optimising immune function?

Athletes are always recommended to ensure their diet is assessed in order to meet their energy demands and to ensure the correct nutrient input to support their immune system. Various dietary components act as important cofactors in immune regulatory pathways and thus significant dietary imbalances can contribute to dysregulation. For this reason, the most useful recommendation is to avoid nutritional deficiencies (which can be achieved with a normal healthy and balanced diet). Since deficiencies will have negative effects, correcting a deficiency will be of benefit. Unfortunately, this has led to a common misconception that taking extra beyond this (e.g. high dose vitamin supplements) will provide further benefit. However, there is little (if any) evidence that consuming extra, above requirements, provides any further benefit if dietary intake is already at the recommended level. Indeed, a limitation with many studies that have suggested additional intake of certain nutrients is beneficial is a failure to determine baseline nutrient status before supplementation (i.e. any benefit observed could simply be caused by the fact that a pre-existing deficiency was corrected, rather than this being caused by the 'apparent' additional intake). Some nutritional practices or supplements (i. e. intakes above that found in a normal diet), however, have good evidence for reducing RTi occurrences and/or severity in athletes but they do usually require weeks to months of supplementation (further details of **some** of these are provided in Table 10.1).

TABLE 10.1 Nutritional supplements and strategies proposed to modulate RTi risk in athletes.

	Benefit when consumed/supplemented? i.e. in those not already deficient/with an adequate diet or nutrient status		Additional comments
	Immune markers (in vitro/ex vivo)	In vivo markers, upper RTi, or other clinically relevant endpoint	
Carbohydrate	☑☑	☐	Research on *in vitro* markers often does not replicate real-life training or competition (e.g. most use fasted exercise). No evidence for CHO supplementation reducing clinically relevant outcomes/endpoints (e.g. RTi).
Antioxidants (e.g. vitamins A, C, E)	☐☐☐	☑☐☐	Some potential benefit of vitamin C in individuals exposed to extreme physical and environmental stressors (e.g. prolonged artic expedition in military; ultra-endurance racing) but unlikely to be of benefit for the vast majority of normal athletes. **Safety/risks?** High intake may block training adaptation.
Vitamin D	☐☐☐	☐☐☐	May be of benefit if athletes are deficient, and prevalence of deficiency is high in many groups of athletes. However, if levels are already adequate then supplementation is unlikely to be of benefit. **Recommendation:** vitamin D status should be checked to determine whether supplementation is required. **Safety/risks?** Excessive intake may be detrimental and harmful.
Multi-nutrient (e.g. multivitamin/minerals).	☑☐☐	☐☐☐	Potential benefit seen in a few small studies with *in vitro* markers but it is not known if this simply reflects increased 'baseline' requirements (relative deficiency). In those without deficiency, no evidence of benefit. **Safety/risks?** Most over-the-counter products (e.g. not exceeding 100% RDA) generally considered safe. Larger doses may be harmful.

(Continued)

Table 10.1 (Cont.)

	Benefit when consumed/supplemented? i.e. in those not already deficient/with an adequate diet or nutrient status		Additional comments
	Immune markers (in vitro/ex vivo)	*In vivo markers, upper RTi, or other clinically relevant endpoint*	
Probiotics	☑☑□	☑☑☑	Many studies have shown benefit with clinically relevant outcomes. Requires time for gut colonization so minimum period of several weeks supplementation needed. Effects are strain specific, and sufficient dose (CFU) needed for efficacy, so not all products are beneficial (recommended to consult with qualified practitioner for best practice). **Safety/risks?** Generally considered safe. Yoghurt versions are dairy products (i.e. not advisable for those with dairy allergy or intolerance).
Bovine colostrum	☑☑□	☑☑☑	Many studies showing benefit with clinically relevant outcomes with ≥ 2 weeks of daily intake (10–20 g/day). **Safety/risks?** Generally considered safe. Contains dairy (lactose and milk proteins). High in IGF-1 content. Most studies show no effect on systemic IGF-1 levels but WADA recommends caution for this reason.
Echinacea	☑☑□	☑☑□	Reasonable evidence for reducing RTi duration in general population but limited research in athletes. **Safety/risks?** Generally considered safe.
Polyphenols	Range: □□□ to ☑☑□ (depending on substance)	Range: □□□ to ☑☑□ (depending on substance)	Reasonable evidence for some compounds (e.g. quercetin) at reducing RTi duration or incidence in a few studies, but findings not replicated in a number of other studies. **Safety/risks?** Generally considered safe, but do have high antioxidant activities so may block training adaptations.

□□□: No evidence of benefit; ☑□□: Limited evidence of benefit; ☑☑□: Reasonable-good evidence of benefit; ☑☑☑: Strong evidence of benefit.
★NOTE: this table is based on evidence of further benefit (or not) above and beyond a normal balanced diet (i.e absence of deficiency).

Acute upper respiratory tract symptoms in athletes – are they always caused by infection?

Several studies have now established that when an athlete presents with 'infective-type' symptoms there is sometimes a low yield rate of confirmed pathogens (i.e. when taking swabs from athletes who report with symptoms of upper RTi, for example one Australian study reported a ~30% confirmation rate). This does not necessarily rule out infectious causes and may relate to the inadequacies of pathogen (especially viral) detection methodologies and this area is rapidly evolving with genetic-based point-of-care equipment becoming more widely available.

It is important to note that the majority of RTis are caused by viral infection. There are over 200 known viruses that cause upper RTi, with the most common being rhinoviruses, coronaviruses, influenza viruses, adenoviruses, parainfluenza viruses, respiratory syncytial viruses and enteroviruses (but most screening methods only test for a select number of the most common pathogens). Therefore, in studies where pathogens were not detected, the athlete could still be infected with one of the other viruses. In addition, some methods (especially in older studies) may have lacked the sensitivity to detect some viruses. For example a much more recent (albeit small) study based in the UK during the winter months (i.e. typical upper RTi season) observed a much higher proportion (82%) of reported illnesses were confirmed by identification of upper RTi-causing pathogens and likewise utilisation of molecular polymerase chain reaction (PCR) based laboratory methods, revealed a high proportion of viral pathogens in an outbreak of upper RTi-type symptoms in recent winter Olympic games.

Having said this, a 'non-infectious hypothesis' proposes that athletes can present with coryzal-type symptoms without evidence of any infective cause. A study of athletic, but non-elite, individuals found a higher incidence of RTi-type symptoms in runners following a marathon (47%) when compared to non-runners (19%) but that this was associated with a positive response in the Allergy Questionnaire for Athletes. The authors proposed that inhalant allergy (16–32% prevalence in highly trained athletes) may have caused the presentation of symptoms that athletes then perceived as upper RTi, when in fact they had no evidence of infection.

Overall this has raised concerns regarding the validity of self-reported upper RTi episodes in athletes. Indeed, discrepancies between physician and laboratory diagnosed upper RTi has also been reported. In some studies infection was found in only half of cases while almost 90% were diagnosed as an infective upper RTi by the assessing physician. One study indicated that the very early part of an infective upper respiratory tract episode (i.e. the first 2 days of symptoms) with either infectious or non-infectious cases were similar but duration and severity of symptoms on subsequent days were greater with an infectious cause. This is one reason why the common symptom scoring methods applied in self-report questionnaire studies usually require symptoms to be present for 2 or more days in order to be counted as an 'episode' and may offer some protection against such limitations. These are important considerations for researchers and practitioners alike.

Other studies have indicated that athletes frequently develop cough following prolonged endurance events and this may be mistakenly taken to indicate the presence of upper RTi, whereas in fact it is more indicative of neuronal airway hyper-sensitivity arising in the airway tract and potentially from the desiccation of the airway surface and accompanying changes in osmolarity (see Chapter 4).

Environmental influences are also likely to be relevant in certain groups of competitive athletes, particularly swimmers who are exposed to chlorine derivatives from pool disinfectants and then inhaling large amounts of air above the water surface. The combination of a high ventilation rate in cold, dry environments may also cause or contribute to the development of RTi-like symptoms in some athletes.

How should I assess an athlete with symptoms of a respiratory tract infection – is it really infection?

Throughout this book, there has been emphasis and focus placed on ensuring that any diagnostic approach involving an athlete utilises the best available investigational strategies. Clinical-based assessment of respiratory symptoms in athletes has notoriously poor predictive power in athletic individuals and as such it is recommended that investigations are used early in any clinical assessment process. The issue, until recently, has been a poor access to test modalities that allow rapid and accurate diagnosis of infection. With the recent advances in point of care molecular diagnostics however there is now the potential to improve the diagnostic assessment process of athletic individuals presenting with upper RTi-type symptoms.

When an athletic individual presents with acute symptoms then it is logical to begin assessment with a thorough history and clinical examination. This process should consider past diagnostic assessments and for example a history of (confirmed) allergic disease, asthma, sinonasal problems and any contributory factors such as gastro-oesophageal reflux. In some cases, an athlete may have previously undergone respiratory screening and thus detailed information regarding airway inflammation and hyper-responsiveness will be already known. It is important to evaluate the severity of symptoms and gauge whether there are features of lower respiratory tract problems (e.g. productive discoloured cough).

Red flags in assessment, such as haemoptysis, sharp chest pain, high fevers, resting breathlessness should warrant urgent medical attention, with a view to immediate blood and radiological investigations.

In most cases however these features won't be apparent and thus a more conservative strategy can be adopted. Investigations with spirometry (i.e. to assess change in FEV_1 and FEV_1/FVC ratio), FeNO (to assess airway inflammation) and blood count for CRP and blood differential white cell count (including eosinophils) are likely to be informative in a testing and treatment strategy.

Nasal and coryzal predominant problems are probably best approached according to details provided in Chapter 8 and asthma type symptoms in Chapters 4–7.

The National Institute for Clinical Excellence (NICE) in 2018 recommended that antibiotics are not given for individuals with acute cough associated with upper respiratory tract infection who were not systemically unwell or at risk of complications (i.e. not clinically vulnerable). In addition, a recent large randomised controlled study showed that a short course of prednisolone in this context was not beneficial and thus is not recommend. Some have recommended illness scores such as the CENTOR score as a means of detecting early risk of progressive infection and other rapid analysis tests such as procalcitonin may prove to be helpful in the future, in this context.

When can an athlete safely 'return to play'?

There are no definitive data to inform the best way to consider a 'right or wrong' answer to when an athlete should 'return to play'. Unfortunately, there are few clear guidelines addressing 'return to play' criteria in respect of respiratory disease. However, it is clear that decisions regarding 'return to play' should be made in cooperation with the athlete's physiotherapist and/or team doctor (as applicable). It is also generally accepted that an athlete with symptoms of infection that are present 'above the neck' only (i.e. as found in upper RTi, e.g. sore throat) can continue training without interruption. However, it is also advised that if infective respiratory symptoms are accompanied by systemic symptoms (e.g. myalgia and fever), then an athlete should abstain from further exercise until their symptoms resolve. Under these circumstances, it is important that athletes are advised that short periods of rest (i.e. 4–5 days) will significantly improve their recovery and have a negligible impact on athletic conditioning. There is no clear evidence of when an athlete can 'return to play' following treatment for community-acquired pneumonia. Series evaluating symptom resolution suggest that up to a month is necessary in some individuals and thus, 'return to play' should be appraised on an individual basis.

On return to sport advise athletes that it can take several weeks to fully recover from a serious infection and that gradual return with performance and load monitoring is essential.

Are there ways to monitor an athlete to detect susceptibility?

Some biomarkers may provide early warnings of increased risk, but it is important to recognise that many so called 'markers' have never been exposed to unblinded prospective validation processes. There is considerable redundancy in the immune system, so measuring a single marker or group of markers does not necessarily correlate with risk of developing upper RTi. If immune biomarkers are to be useful in determining risk, markers which are 'clinically relevant' must be selected.

Saliva secretory immunoglobulin A (IgA) is commonly used as it is non-invasive and there is some data showing an association exists between this marker and upper

RTi risk. However, there is massive variability in this marker between individuals and to be of practical benefit to athletes in providing 'early warning' information, regular monitoring and measurements are required with rapid availability of results (which is not always feasible). Furthermore, saliva markers may be invalidated if samples are contaminated with blood (even in minute quantities that cannot be detected by visual inspection of samples). For salivary IgA, this problem can be avoided by selecting an assay that is specific to the secretory IgA (as this is not found in blood, only mucosal secretions). Practitioners should be aware of this, however and ensure they select an appropriate method (note, many POC-type/ rapid tests marketed for athletes to test salivary IgA are not specific to secretory IgA and may produce inaccurate results due to salivary blood contamination). In addition to biomarkers, training diaries, mood states, sleep patterns, diet logs, exercising (and resting) heart rate and performance can all be used to help to identify if an athlete does not match up to their 'normal' profile and might be at risk of subsequent infection. It is important to note that for any measure it is important to first establish the normal (healthy) baseline profile for the athlete.

Conclusion

Respiratory tract infection is a major issue in athlete health and should be an area of focus and concern for any healthcare team or system concerned with athlete welfare. There are several relevant and unique factors that make athletes susceptible to infection and when infection does occur it can significantly impact training and performance. Strategies should be used to minimise risk and exposure to infection, and when upper RTi-type symptoms do occur then it is essential that logical clinical assessment allied with rapid access to the best diagnostic tests is recognised as key to ensuring best outcome for the athlete.

OVERALL RECOMMENDATIONS TO MINIMISE INFECTION RISK IN ATHLETES

- Try to avoid sick people, particularly in the autumn–winter.
- Ensure good hand hygiene and appropriate vaccination.
- Avoid self-inoculation by touching the eyes, nose and mouth.
- Do not train or compete with 'below-the-neck' symptoms.
- Monitor and manage all forms of stress including physical and psychosocial.
- Carefully manage increments in training stress.
- Replace overly long training sessions with more frequent spike sessions.
- Plan recovery or adaptation week every second or third week.
- Aim for at least 7 h sleep each night.
- Eat a well-balanced diet and avoid chronic low energy availability.

Multiple-choice questions

1.   Which of the following may contribute to increased RTi risk in athletes?

   (A)   Nutritional deficiency
   (B)   Psychological stress
   (C)   Sudden increase in training load (e.g. intensity and duration)
   (D)   Long-haul travel for competition
   (E)   All of the above

2.   Sleeping less than 6 h per night is associated with a _____-fold increase in susceptibility to the common cold?

   (A)   0.5
   (B)   2
   (C)   3
   (D)   4
   (E)   6

3.   Antibiotics are an effective treatment for most RTis:

   ●   True
   ●   False

4.   In the Northern Hemisphere, RTi incidence is higher in the winter

   ●   True
   ●   False

5.   Single biomarkers of immune status are not always useful for predicting risk of RTi in athletes because:

   (A)   The immune system is not involved in protecting against RTis
   (B)   There is considerable redundancy in the immune system, so a single marker may not reflect overall ability of the immune system to fight RTi-causing pathogens
   (C)   The technology is currently not available to measure biomarkers accurately
   (D)   They cannot provide results quickly enough
   (E)   It is too difficult to diagnose RTi

Online resources

Hand washing steps: www.icliniq.com/articles/healthy-living-wellness-and-prevention/hand-washing-steps

Key reading

Albers R, Bourdet-Sicard R, Braun D, Calder PC, Herz U, Lambert Cet al. (2013). Monitoring immune modulation by nutrition in the general population: identifying and substantiating effects on human health. *British Journal of Nutrition*, 110(Suppl 2):S1–S30.

Cunniffe B, Griffiths H, Proctor W, Davies B, Baker JS, Jones KP. Mucosal immunity and illness incidence in elite rugby union players across a season. *Med Sci Sports Exerc*, 2011;43 (3):388–397. doi:10.1249/MSS.0b013e3181ef9d6b.

Davison G, Kehaya C, Jones AW (2016). Nutritional and Physical Activity Interventions to Improve Immunity. *American Journal of Lifestyle Medicine*, 10(3): 152–169. doi:10.1177/1559827614557773.

Gleeson M, Walsh NP (2012). The BASES expert statement on exercise, immunity, and infection. *Journal of Sports Sciences*, 30(3):321–324.

Hellard P, Avalos M, Guimaraes F, Toussaint J-F, Pyne DB. Training-related risk of common illnesses in elite swimmers over a 4-yr period. *Med Sci Sports Exerc*, 2015;47 (4):698–707. doi:10.1249/MSS.0000000000000461.

Keaney LC, Kilding AE, Merien F, Dulson DK. Keeping Athletes Healthy at the 2020 Tokyo Summer Games: Considerations and Illness Prevention Strategies. *Front Physiol*, 2019;10. doi:10.3389/fphys.2019.00426.

Pyne DB, Hopkins WG, Batterham AM, Gleeson M, Fricker PA (2005). Characterising the individual performance responses to mild illness in international swimmers. *Br J Sports Med*, 39(10):752–756.

Svendsen IS, Taylor IM, Tønnessen E, Bahr R, Gleeson M. Training-related and competition-related risk factors for respiratory tract and gastrointestinal infections in elite cross-country skiers. *Br J Sports Med*, 2016;50(13):809–815. doi:10.1136/bjsports-2015-095398.

Walsh NP. Recommendations to maintain immune health in athletes. *Eur J Sport Sci*, 2018;18(6):820–831. doi:10.1080/17461391.2018.1449895.

Williams NC, Killer SC, Svendsen IS, Jones AW. Immune nutrition and exercise: Narrative review and practical recommendations. *Eur J Sport Sci*, 2019;19(1):49–61. doi:10.1080/17461391.2018.1490458.

Answers: 1 (E), 2 (D), 3 False, 4 True, 5 (B)

11

BREATHING PATTERN DISORDERS IN ATHLETES

John W. Dickinson and Anna Boniface

Overview

This chapter will cover:

- Definition of a breathing pattern disorder.
- Explanation of how athletes develop breathing pattern disorders.
- What the performance implications are for an athlete with a breathing pattern disorder.
- How to detect and diagnose breathing pattern disorders in athletes.
- What therapy is available for athletes with breathing pattern disorders.

Introduction

Exercise and sport is a physiological stressor, particularly at high intensity. As discussed in Chapter 1, respiration is an automatic process, but it can be influenced by our conscious control. This can result in activation of accessory respiratory muscles, which can lead to insufficient movement of the chest wall, reduced tidal volumes, increased breathing frequency and the development of both respiratory and non-respiratory symptoms (See Table 11.1). This array of symptoms can be described as dysfunctional breathing, or a breathing pattern disorder (BPD). The purpose of this chapter is to discuss BPD in athletes during exercise.

There are several causes that can contribute to BPD, which are a mixture of physiological, psychological, social and environmental triggers (Table 11.2). With persistent exposure to these triggers hyper-arousal of the nervous system can occur. Signs and symptoms such as reduced tolerance and increased levels of dyspnoea become habitual through the brain associating past emotional experiences with changes in breathing.

TABLE 11.1 Symptoms and signs of BPD during exercise

Respiratory symptoms	Respiratory signs
• Breathlessness disproportionate to activity • Chest tightness • Unable to take a deep breath • Wheeze on inspiration (linked to exercise induced laryngeal obstruction – see Chapter 9)	• Upper chest breathing dominance • Asynchrony between abdomen and chest movement • Hyperinflated chest (BradCliff Angle Tests) • Rapid, shallow or irregular breathing pattern during exercise (can also occur at rest) • Difficulty synching breathing with talking and/or movement cadence. • Throat clearing/habitual coughing
Musculoskeletal symptoms	**Musculoskeletal signs**
• Neck, shoulder, upper back pain and tension • Peripheral muscle pain, burning and fatigue • Jaw tension	• Recruitment of upper chest muscles • Imbalance in abdominal and back muscles • Abdominal splinting • Pelvic floor weakness • Rounded/hunched shoulder posture
Neurological symptoms	**Other signs and symptoms**
• Blurred vision • Brain Fog • Headaches • Numbness • Tingling hands/ pins and needles • Disorientated • Fainting	• Frequent yawning or sighing • Stomach upset/ bladder/bowel problems • Anxious • Stressed
Cardiovascular symptoms	
• Chest pain • Palpations • Relatively high heart rate for the exercise work • Reduced SaO_2 during exercise	

Source: adapted from Bradley and Clifton Smith (2005)

BPDs vary in severity and type. Hyperventilation syndrome (HVS) is at the severe end of the spectrum. An athlete will describe symptoms of air hunger and feelings of suffocation. These symptoms are usually at rest with frequent yawning, sighing and erratic breathing patterns. In HVS, chemoreceptors have increased sensitisation to reduced levels of carbon dioxide (pCO2). Increased levels of pCO2 and pH stimulate the drive to breathe to maintain ventilation (e.g. the urge to breathe when swimming underwater). In HVS, the urge to breathe will occur with normal pCO_2 levels due to a reduced tolerance. Most BPDs occur in the absence of hypocapnia where symptoms such as chest tightness are caused by dynamic hyperinflation from incomplete exhalation.

TABLE 11.2 Causes of breathing pattern disorders

Biomechanical	Cultural
• Postural abnormalities e.g. Scoliosis • Excess upper limb movement e.g. Swimmers • Chronic mouth breathing e.g. from nasal congestion • Congenital • Abnormal movement patterns • Braced postures e.g. time trial position in cycling	• Breathing in for aesthetics e.g. in gymnastics • Tight restrictive clothing
Psychological	**Physiological**
• Anxiety & panic disorder • Stress • Type A personality • Suppressed emotions e.g. anger • History of abuse • Learnt response • Anticipation • Depression • Pain • Phobias • Mental tasks with sustained concentration and boredom	• Lung disease • Metabolic disease • Allergies • Diet e.g. intolerances causing bloating, hypoglycaemia. • Speech/laughter • Chronic low grade fever • Exercise
	Biochemical
	• Drugs – recreational, caffeine, aspirin • Hormones – raised progesterone levels during the menstrual cycle. Hormonal changes during the menopause.
	Environmental
	• Heat • Altitude • Humidity

It is common for those with respiratory conditions such as asthma to experience BPD, especially during exercise. If a respiratory condition (e.g. asthma) is detected, it's important athletes symptoms and airway health are appropriately managed through the optimisation of inhaled therapies in the first instance (see Chapters 4–8). However, if respiratory disease or other organic causes of symptoms have been excluded and/or appropriately managed, breathing pattern retraining may be beneficial.

WHAT IS A NORMAL BREATHING PATTERN?

Normal breathing at rest should be:

- Quiet and relaxed.
- Through the nose and not the mouth, which should stay closed.
- Shoulders and upper chest should stay still with no accessory muscle use.
- Abdominal ribcage movements using the lower intercostal muscles and the diaphragm.
- Expiration passive and relaxed.
- Rate of 8–18 breaths per minute.
- Inspiration to expiration ratio approximately 1:2.
- Smooth and rhythmical.

Changes during exercise

Breathing needs to change during exercise to meet metabolic demands. As exertion increases changes seen include:

- Increase in rate and depth of breathing.
- Gradual transition from nose to mouth breathing.
- Increased upper chest expansion and more forceful inspiration required with accessory muscle recruitment (external intercostals, scalenes, sternocleidomastoid, pectoralis minor).
- Active expiration with increased abdominal and internal intercostal muscle use.

FORMS OF BREATHING PATTERN DISORDER

Excessive accessory respiratory muscle recruitment and shoulder activation *or* excessive accessory muscle use: Characterised by limited lateral movement of abdominal rib cage and along with stiff or raised shoulders, sometimes rounded. Results in limited movement of rib cage limiting tidal volume, with athlete having to increase breathing frequency in an attempt to achieve desired minute ventilation.

Asynchrony between abdominal and chest movement: Characterised by abdomen moving significantly before chest wall moves. Results in bi-phasic inspiratory flow and reduced tidal volume. Athlete has to increase breathing frequency in order to achieve required minute ventilation.

Hyperventilation: Movement of abdomen and chest in synchronisation and no obvious over activation of respiratory accessory muscles, however athlete over breathing for the work they performing

What are the performance implications of BPD during exercise?

An athlete with BPD may be able to train and compete but their performance is likely to be compromised. BPD can result in increased respiratory muscle work, reduction in arterial oxygen saturation (SaO_2), prolonged recovery from intermittent exercise and early cessation of high-intensity exercise. **It is common for coaches to perceive the poor performance resulting from BPD to be due to lack of physical conditioning or effort.**

Athletes who have a BPD may be able to perform at a low-moderate exercise intensity without symptoms or a reduction in performance, however when exercise intensity increases they begin to experience significant symptoms and their performance is adversely affected.

This occurs from reduced chest wall movements reducing tidal volume (volume of air per breath). To compensate for this, breath frequency will increase creating increased work on the respiratory muscles. This increases the relative energy cost of ventilation and compromises oxygen diffusion, all of which may result in reduced performance and potential early cessation of exercise.

From a mechanical perspective, a BPD results in incomplete inhalation and 'dynamic hyperinflation'. This can cause an airflow reduction and alveolar dead space from the hyperinflation compressing adjacent airways and capillaries. Mechanically, BPD can cause the diaphragm to be flattened. This contributes to upper chest breathing, accessory muscle use and premature muscle fatigue.

As work of breathing increases, oxygenated blood is diverted away from the peripheral muscles towards the diaphragm to prioritise breathing in means of a protection system. This 'blood stealing' or respiratory metaboreflex can occur during intensive exercise. An athlete with a BPD may experience a shift of breathing mechanics at lower intensities causing an earlier onset of respiratory metaboreflex compared to the athlete without a BPD.

What is the prevalence of BPD in athletes?

There are currently no standardised assessments that allow for a clear diagnosis of BPD. In the majority of cases, BPD diagnosis is based on clinical signs and symptoms, and the exclusion of cardiopulmonary and metabolic disease. From our experience, BPD is often present in high achieving athletes, although there is no published report of BPD in athletes. Future work is required to develop standardised methods to diagnose BPD and report on the prevalence of the condition across all sports.

Despite the prevalence of BPD is unknown, we do know that many athletes with symptoms of BPD (Table 11.1) can be incorrectly diagnosed with exercise-induced bronchoconstriction (EIB; see Chapter 5). Athletes incorrectly diagnosed with EIB will not experience a significant reduction from inhaler therapy (e.g. short acting β_2-Agonist) due to absence of bronchoconstriction. To reduce the misdiagnosis of BPD as EIB objective airway assessments should be utilised with athletes that have suspected BPD to either rule in or rule out asthma-related conditions (Chapter 5). Practitioners should also consider athletes may experience both EIB and BPD. BPD may occur in those athletes with exercise induced laryngeal obstruction (see Chapter 9). It is not clear whether the BPD leads to the development of EILO, or whether the EILO drives the athlete to develop a BPD.

How do I understand the athlete's symptoms and perceived performance limitations?

The initial athlete interaction is essential to gain an understanding of their background, symptoms and their perception of how it impacts their performance. It is good practice to get to know the athlete and build rapport with them in the early stages. Key information to obtain includes past medical history, previous diagnosis of respiratory, cardiovascular or metabolic disease, prescribed medication, training and competition schedule, symptoms and any previous strategies they have used to manage them.

CONSIDERATIONS TO UNDERSTANDING THE ATHLETE'S SYMPTOMS AND PERCEIVED LIMITATIONS

What are the athletes main symptoms and perceived performance implications?

- Breathlessness – What does their breathing feel like? Scoring of severity using the Modified Borg Scale.
- Cough – Dry, productive, intractable.
- Chest tightness – Location – upper or lower chest?
- Symptom onset – timing, triggers, are they worse with exercise? Do they improve when they stop exercising? How long do they take to get better? Do they occur at rest?
- Limitations to performance – how does it impact their performance? Does it stop them training or competing?

Lifestyle factors

- Sleep – quality, weekly average, do they feel refreshed on waking?
- Work/studying, social/family commitments, sponsor/funding pressures – is the athlete feeling stressed?
- Caffeine intake.
- Smoking status.
- Recreational drug use.
- Relaxation time.

Sport-specific:

- Current level – club, regional, national, international.
- Years in the sport.
- Weekly training schedule (volume, intensity).
- Current level of fitness.
- Coach.
- Target competitions and goals.

Are there any questionnaires that can be included in the diagnosis of BPD?

Currently, there are no questionnaires specific to BPD in athletes, however, validated questionnaires and scales, such as Nijmegen and Borg scale can be used to gain an appreciation of respiratory symptoms and current situation.

The Nijmegen Questionnaire is primarily designed to help identify individuals with hyperventilation syndrome. It is not validated for exercise and therefore should only be used for an athlete to score there symptoms at rest rather than specifically related to exercise. The questionnaire scores a range of symptoms from stress, difficulty in breathing and symptoms of hypocapnia. Scores of above 23 are indicative of hyperventilation syndrome. Important to note an athlete may still have BPD can still exist without positive Nijmegen score.

The Brompton Breathing Pattern Assessment Tool (BPAT) has been designed to assess for BPD in patients with and without the diagnosis of asthma. It involves assessing a patient at rest for 1 minute and objectively scoring 7 components of their breathing pattern. This will give a score that can be used to detect a BPD.

What objective assessments are available to assess athletes for BPD?

We can use objective observations and assessments to help identify and characterise BPD. There are no standardised assessments to identify BPD in athletes. However, using a combination of assessments at rest and during exercise can help the practitioner and athlete understand and characterise the BPD.

Observe resting breathing pattern

A simple method is to observe the athletes breathing pattern at rest. The athlete should ideally be unaware when you are observing their breathing pattern, therefore observing can be taken subtly when taking the athletes pulse or when they are filling in a questionnaire. When observing breathing rate you should look for the following:

- Resting respiratory rate (normal rate between 8–18 breathes per minute).
- Nose or mouth breather.
- Predominately chest or abdomen movements.
- Regular or irregular breathing pattern.
- Accessory muscle activation.
- Abdominal or pelvic splinting.
- Breath holding.
- Sighing, yawing, throat clearing and coughing.
- Difficulty timing breathing with talking.

What musculoskeletal and postural assessments should I consider?

Musculoskeletal and postural problems can both contribute to and result from a BPD (Table 11.3). If hypocapnia and respiratory alkalosis is present it can increase muscle tone and reduce blood flow to muscles which can result in trigger points. Furthermore, dynamic hyperinflation and upper chest breathing alter the diaphragm length-tension relationship and overuse of the accessory muscles. This can cause postural imbalances, weaken core stability muscles and increase spinal rigidity.

However, it's important to consider that an athlete's posture or underlying musculoskeletal issues can impact their breathing mechanics. Postural stability and respiration play a dual role in pressure regulation. Impairments from postural abnormalities or musculoskeletal conditions may alter muscle recruitment and optimal alinement.

What cardio-pulmonary assessments should I consider?

It is common for athletes with BPD to present within healthy boundaries when they undergo clinical cardio-pulmonary assessments. However, it is recommended athletes reporting respiratory symptoms undergo the following investigations in

TABLE 11.3 Musculoskeletal areas to consider during BPD assessment

Posture	• Assess posture in lying, sitting, standing. • Consider different posture types e.g. lordotic, sway back posture, pelvic tilting (lateral, anterior and posterior). • Assess sporting postures, particularly if the athlete is in sustained or repetitive postures e.g. aerodynamic position in time trial cycling. • Discussion of work/study ergonomics. • Assessment of muscle imbalances. • Bracing of abdominal muscles.
Core stability	• Assess activation spinal stabilisation muscles such as pelvic floor and transverse abdominus. • Functional activities to establish neuromuscular control e.g. bridging, sitting on a gym ball, single leg squat and sports specific movements.
Pain	• Body chart for areas of pain. • Pain score.
Spinal, thoracic and shoulder girdle mobility	• Active and passive range of movement. • Accessory movements of spine, ribs and shoulder.
Spinal and thoracic structure	• Spinal deformities – scoliosis, kyphosis, kypho-scolosis. • Chest wall deformities – pectus carinatum, pectus exvacatum.
Muscle strength, length and tension	• Assessment of muscle imbalances through muscle strength and length of opposing postural muscle groups. • Palpation for areas of muscle tension and trigger point.

order to rule in or out any cardio-pulmonary disease that may be the underlying cause of the respiratory symptoms (Table 11.4).

The list in Table 11.4 is not exhaustive and where indicated other assessments can be added (e.g. allergy skin prick test). It is likely that if the athlete has BPD all of the above tests will present with normative boundaries and a further exercise challenge (see below) should be considered. However, if the above assessments indicate a potential issue (e.g. EIB) this should be dealt with initially and appropriate monitoring of athlete should take place once they have initiated therapy. If the respiratory symptoms persist despite adequate control of co-existing conditions then the athlete should undergo exercise challenge (see below) to investigate for BPD.

How do you use an exercise challenge to detect BPD?

Most athletes who report symptoms of BPD usually report that they occur during high-intensity exercise. Therefore, the purpose of any exercise challenge exploring BPD should incorporate a form of exercise that replicates when the athletes experience their symptoms. **Utilising a high-intensity repeated sprint protocol has been shown to be effective in evidencing the ability of an athlete to recover and control breathing in between efforts.** Utilising a challenge that involves repeated high-intensity efforts lasting approximately 30–60 seconds with a self-selected recovery up to 30 seconds between sprints has been used previously to investigate for BPD in elite athletes.

When designing the exercise challenge consider when the athlete reports their symptoms, what environment triggers their symptoms and the activity the symptoms occur in. Aim to have the athlete complete 5 to 15 repeated efforts (lasting up 60 s for each effort) depending on the athlete's fitness and severity of their symptoms. The intensity of the sprints should be close to maximal but the athlete needs to be reminded to pace themselves, to an extent, so they can complete the set number of sprints. The challenge only needs to continue until the athlete reports

TABLE 11.4 Cardio-pulmonary assessments to consider

Respiratory	Baseline spirometry, fractional exhaled nitric oxide concentration (FeNo), airway challenge for EIB (see Chapter 5), chest X-ray. If inspiratory wheeze reported athletes may undergo investigations for EILO (see Chapter 10).
Bloods	Full blood count (anaemia, eosinophilia), Immunoglobins.
Cardiology	Echo, stress tests, electro cardiogram (ECG).
Exercise	Cardiopulmonary exercise testing (CPET; see Chapter 1).

their symptoms are occurring. A familiarisation to the challenge can take place but this is not always possible in an applied setting.

During the challenge record heart rate at the end of each sprint along with the athlete's perception of breathlessness via the modified Borg Scale. The athlete can also wear a pulse oximeter to record peripheral capillary oxygen saturation (SpO_2). Lateral movement of the lower rib cage and assessing synchrony between the chest and the abdomen are specific areas to observe. It is best practice to video the athletes breathing pattern. The video footage is best take directly after the final effort and should be shot while the athlete stationary. Take footage from the athletes hips to their neck from behind them and from the side. Ten to twenty seconds from each position should be sufficient for analysis. The observations and video can be used to assess the athlete for BPD and are valuable to assist clinical reasoning of a BPD and help devise the athlete's treatment plan.

EMERGING NON-INVASIVE METHODS TO MONITOR BREATHING PATTERN

Opto-electronic plethysmography

Opto-electronic plethysmography (OEP) is a method to evaluate ventilation and chest and abdomen wall movements through an external measurement of the chest wall surface motion. A number of small reflective markers are placed on the thoraco-abdominal surface. A system for human motion analysis measures the three-dimensional coordinates of these markers and the enclosed volume is computed by connecting the points to form triangles. From OEP the chest and abdomen can be split into three different compartments: pulmonary rib cage (RCp), abdominal rib cage (RCa), and the abdomen (AB). This model is the most appropriate for the study of chest wall kinematics in the majority of conditions, including exercise. The downside of the OEP is that it is time consuming, has to take place in a biomechanics laboratory and requires skilled technicians.

Structured light plethysmography

Structured light plethysmography (SLP) technology is a non-invasive method for measuring chest and abdominal wall movement. A checkerboard pattern of light is projected from a light projector onto the chest of an individual. Movements of the grid are viewed by two digital cameras, digitalised, and processed to form a 3D model and can be interrogated to assess lung function. SLP is simple to use, cost effective, is self-calibrating. SLP also needs to take place in an area with limited light exposure to allow the device to track the grid movement. The downside to SLP is that it only measures a set area (front) of the chest and abdomen and it cannot be used during exercise. However, it is possible to take SLP measurements pre and post exercise.

Wearable technology

Development of wearable technology may mean we are able to measure movements of the chest and abdomen wall in field based settings. This form of technology is still under development and the ideas focus around development of garments that have embedded sensors to track movements. This method of measuring chest and abdomen wall movements will help provide real time feedback to the athlete regarding their current breathing performance and aid practitioners in detecting and treating BPD.

What therapy can be used to reduce or eliminate BPD?

In the initial stages, reassurance and education are essential. It should be emphasised that athlete's respiratory symptoms can be reduced/eliminated and breathing pattern can be improved. Educating the athlete, especially through discussion of your assessment and showing them video feedback will increase their awareness of their breathing mechanics and help gain an understanding of the underlying cause of their symptoms.

This should be followed by an explanation of their treatment plan and setting appropriate goals with the athlete. There is no set time limit for breathing retraining to significantly improve their symptoms. It can vary between days and months before they will notice any changes. Reassurance that responses to retraining are individualised and feelings of discomfort in the initial stages may occur but are not usually harmful.

Although not all athletes experience symptoms at rest, breathing retraining should begin by building general awareness of their current breathing pattern and start correcting breathing mechanics at rest prior to shifting the focus towards more sports specific, functional exercises (see Figure 11.1).

What does the progression of breathing pattern training involve?

The athlete should be started in beach pose (see Figure 11.2) to retrain and build awareness of a diaphragmatic breathing pattern. Initially allow the athlete to gain awareness of their breathing pattern e.g. whether they breathe from their chest or abdomen, if they breathe from their mouth or nose, or if they breathe slow or fast. Once they are aware of their current breathing pattern, instruct them to breathe softly and rhythmical through their nose. By ensuring they are relaxed, instruct them to breathe from their abdomen, expanding their lower rib cage, while minimising upper chest movements (see Figure 11.3). A useful online tutorial for building breathing awareness and instructions for correcting breathing mechanics at rest can be found at www.breathestudy.co.uk. See Table 11.5 below for further cues and for troubleshooting common problems in breathing retraining.

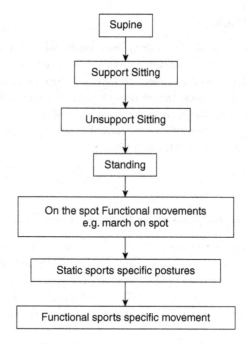

FIGURE 11.1 Progression of breathing pattern retraining positions and movements.

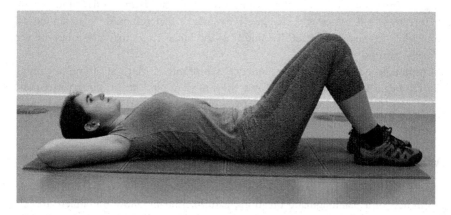

FIGURE 11.2 Beach pose.

When the athlete can comfortably breathe in the beach pose for 5 minutes, they can be progressed into sitting, standing (Figures 11.4 and 11.5), more challenging postures (Figures 11.6 and 11.7). Functional movements can be added that may include actions such as standing on the spot and swing arms to mimic arm action during running. Throughout all exercises the athlete should focus on the fundamental breathing pattern movements encouraged during the supine, seated and standing exercises.

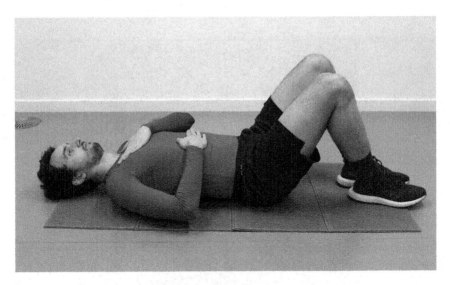

FIGURE 11.3 Laying down hands on abdomen and chest.

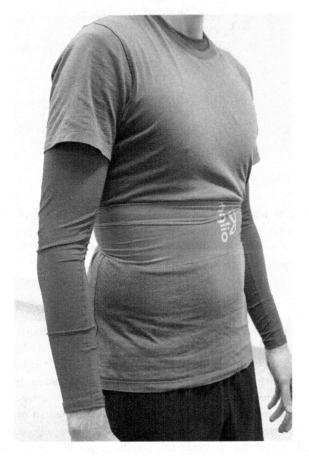

FIGURE 11.4 Standing with Theraband.

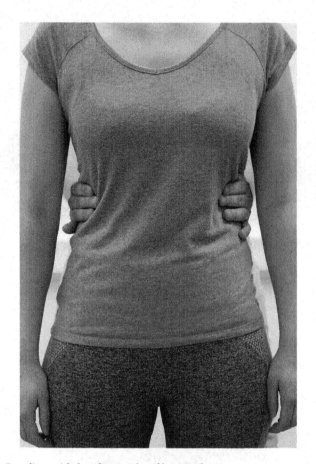

FIGURE 11.5 Standing with hands on side of lower ribs.

The athlete should focus on smooth breathing action focusing on initiating each breath in with outward movements (laterally, horizontally and vertically) of lower ribs and abdomen and with deeper breathes finally leading to expansion of the upper chest. Athletes should be encouraged to progress these exercises to make them as functional and sport-specific as possible. For example a cyclist can progress their breathing pattern training to executing the breathing pattern while holding cycling posture on their bike.

Each breathing exercise should be performed for at least 2 minutes a day. Athletes may also wish to use bands or have a partner place hands around the lower ribs to help with proprioception of the breath initiation (Figures 11.4 and 11.5). If athletes use a breathing aid (e.g. hands on side of ribs) they should use the aid for two minutes and then perform the breathing exercise without the aid for two – three minutes. **It can be helpful to video the breathing exercise so the athlete can observe it afterwards and analyse their technique.** Athletes should not progress their breathing exercises until they are able to consistently breathe as described above for a 2 minutes period on two consecutive days.

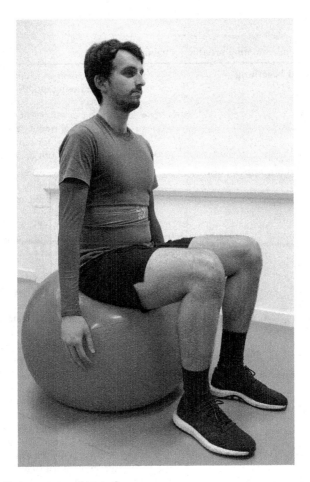

FIGURE 11.6 Sitting on unstable surface.

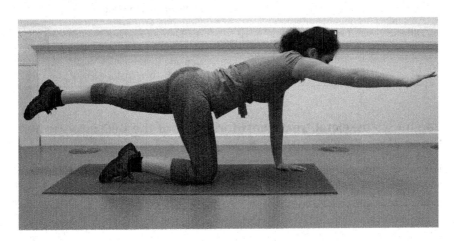

FIGURE 11.7 Breathing pattern exercise while holding a superman pose.

TABLE 11.5 Trouble shooting breathing retraining

Difficultly nasal breathing	• Encouragement of keeping mouth closed and using mouth taping where appropriate. • Education of soft, silent breathing. • Teaching nasal rinsing techniques if appropriate (e.g. for sinus congestion encouraging mouth breathing).
Difficultly reducing upper chest breathing	• Using beach pose position. • Verbal cues of relaxing the shoulders, keeping the chest still and breathing from the stomach. • Proprioceptive feedback through gentle pressure applied to the upper chest e.g. with a bag of sugar or the clinicians hands. • Reducing excess shoulder movement through the clinician restricting excess shoulder girdle elevation. • Emphasis on relaxation strategies. • Musculoskeletal treatment of accessory muscles or restrictions in the shoulder girdle/thorax as appropriate.
Difficultly abdominal breathing	• Cue the athlete to place their hands on their abdomen and cough – cue them to breathe from this area. • Proprioceptive feedback- placing hands on the side of the lower ribs or abdomen, using Kinesiology tape or a resistance band across the diaphragm for tactile stimulus/visual aid.
Hyperventilation • Incomplete exhalation and breath stacking • Air hunger/feelings of suffocation • Difficultly with breathing rhythm, speed and depth	• Pursed lipped breathing can be taught to promote lengthened expiration and reduce respiratory rate. • Counting or using a metronome to aid rhythmical breathing. • Controlled pauses at the end of expiration and incorporating breath holds can be used when hypocapnia is suspected.

Can musculoskeletal treatments form part of the BPD intervention therapy?

Following a musculoskeletal assessment, problems that are related to the athletes BPD should be addressed. As discussed previously, musculoskeletal disorders and poor posture can either contribute or be a result of a BPD. Table 11.6 shows the treatment areas to consider.

TABLE 11.6 Musculoskeletal treatment options for athletes with BPD

Posture	• Postural awareness education. • Stretching of shortened muscles and strengthening of lengthened weak muscles. • Core stability and Pilates. • Spinal mobility. • Ergonomic advice and assessment (e.g. work and studying set up, carrying bags, driving set up). • Sporting equipment adjustments (e.g. bike fit). • Taping techniques for proprioceptive feedback on postural retraining.
Spinal mobility	• Spinal mobility exercises. • Manual therapy for the spine and ribs. • Soft tissue mobilisation and massage.
Core and spinal stability	• Exercises targeted at key stability muscles such as pelvic floor, multifidis and transverse abdominus.
Pain	• Discussion with medical professionals for pain optimisation. • Acupuncture. • Manual therapy and soft tissue mobilisation. • Pain education.

Can inspiratory muscle training help athletes overcome BPD?

A limitation of the above breathing training is that it doesn't necessarily challenge the athlete to practice breathing at a similar intensity to their sport. A solution to this is to use inspiratory muscle training (IMT). Chapter 12 goes into greater detail on how to use IMT with a breathing training programme. It has been demonstrated to previously be useful for athletes with BPD and EILO. During this IMT training, the athlete is instructed to breathe in hard and fast thus replicating inspiratory manoeuvres similar to high-intensity exercise. While completing the IMT it is paramount the athlete focuses on the quality of their breathing pattern as outlined above. They are encouraged to initiate the breath through expansion of lower ribcage and abdomen with the upper rib cage expanding smoothly until the athlete completes the inspiratory phase reaching their total lung capacity (TLC). Once the athlete reaches TLC the following exhalation should be smooth, controlled and relaxed, lasting between 5–10 seconds. The athlete should aim to complete 30 breathes during an IMT session.

Athletes engaging in IMT for their BPD should be encouraged to focus on the quality of their breathing pattern rather than obsess about the IMT resistance. A common mistake by athletes using IMT as part of their breathing training is they increase the IMT resistance too much, which results in them adopting inappropriate breathing patterns.

Once the athlete is comfortable perming IMT in an upright stationary position they can progress to performing IMT holding more functional postures and movements. If athletes do progress their IMT to functional movements consider reducing the resistance of the device to ensure the quality of the breathing pattern is not compromised.

LIFESTYLE FACTORS TO DISCUSS WITH ATHLETE WHO HAS BPD

Rest and sleep

- Identify any causes of sleep disturbances (e.g. snoring partner).
- Commit the athlete to a sleep plan.
- Sleep hygiene strategies (e.g. reduce mental stimulating activities before sleep – blue light exposure, TV; avoid late training sessions; reduce caffeine intake; and reduce fluid intake before bed).
- Aim for a weekly average sleep target of over 8 hours.
- Management strategies for travel and changes in time zones.

Nutrition

- Ensure consistent energy and nutritional intake throughout the day to avoid fluctuating glucose levels.
- Breakfast is essential and encourage regular eating every 3 hours.
- Referral to a dietician if required

Relaxation techniques

- Establish both mental and physical relaxation strategies.
- A quiet, warm and comfortable environment to practice relaxation.
- Using appropriate adjuncts such as meditation apps.

Use in conjunction with breathing techniques.

Psychological factors

An athlete's psychology can be significant contributing factor to a BPD and often the root cause to their symptoms. Anxiety, fear and stress can overstimulate the autonomic nervous system causing physiological changes to breathing that have been discussed throughout the chapter.

It is not uncommon for athletes to experience pre-competition anxiety and to feel out of control about their performance through issues such as illness or injury. Negative experiences, such as a severe injury during their sport can also evoke fearful emotions which can be a potential trigger for abnormal breathing patterns.

It is essential to discuss with the athlete about any triggers, fear or anxiety around their sport. Using screening tools such as the Patient Health

Questionnaire – 9 or Generalised Anxiety Disorder test can be used but are not specific to athletes.

If psychological issues are established, referral to a sports psychologist is useful. Strategies for managing fear, stress and anxiety need to be put in place to promote relaxation, increase coping and reduce their emotional triggers. Common strategies include visualisation, positive self-talk and relaxation techniques in combination with breathing exercises, which can also be utilised during the athlete's warm-up routine.

Once an athlete has appropriately managed their BPD can it ever return?

An athlete who has had BPD and subsequently overcome it may still in frequently experience symptoms. Athletes who have overcome BPD report significant reduction in respiratory symptoms, however they do note that there are occasions where they experience symptoms. Most athletes are able to notice the early signs of the development of a dysfunctional breathing pattern and can use their experience of their breathing pattern training to revert to an efficient breathing pattern before their symptoms escalate. However, there are occasions where BPD may resurface after a period of time (months) of exercising symptom free. This can happen for a number of reasons, including:

- Athlete has disengaged with the breathing pattern training once BPD symptoms are not present anymore.
- Injury which either directly or indirectly impact on athlete posture or breathing pattern.
- Stress/anxiety related to a specific competition or performance.
- Athlete competes/trains in an environment they don't like (e.g. very hot or cold, windy).

How can an athlete reduce the chances of BPD reoccurring?

Once an athlete has overcome their BPD they should aim to continue to engage with the breathing pattern training programme. However, they do not need to continue to perform the exercises on a daily basis. They should look to perform a lighter version of the breathing training programme that they engage with three to four times a week. This will enable them to continue to progress their ability to breathing in a variety of postures and better prepare them for days when they are challenged by either the environment or a stressful situation.

CASE STUDY

26-year-old elite female swimmer struggling to complete high-intensity swimming sessions. Her symptoms during high-intensity swimming included shortness of breath, tight chest, air hunger, light headed. Using inhaled asthma therapy (salbutamol) did not resolve her symptoms. Within 5 minutes of finishing swimming session symptoms had resolved. Her symptoms were negatively impacting on her ability to complete high-intensity training sessions and her coach was beginning to think she would not be able to complete the training required to compete at the highest level. Investigations for cardio-respiratory disease did not identify an underlying cause for the symptoms. Baseline spirometry was normal and remained so following specific exercise challenges for BPD (10 × 100 m with self-determined recovery up to 30 s). Directly following the challenge swimmers breathing pattern was recorded and it was clear she had an asynchronic breathing pattern. Swimmer was reassured about her symptoms and her BPD explained. She initiated a training programme that included education, breathing pattern technique and IMT. She conducted the sessions on a daily basis prior to engaging with her swimming pre-pool routine. Her progressed was monitored by a therapist on a weekly basis. A follow-up assessment was conducted 6 weeks following initiation of the breathing training programme. At this point her breathing pattern was visibly improved, the swimmers symptoms had significantly reduced and she was able to complete all high-intensity training without having to modify it for respiratory symptoms. The swimmer was advised to continue to be mindful of their breathing pattern to avoid reverting back to a dysfunctional pattern.

Conclusion

Breathing pattern disorders are frequently encountered in athletes; however, the prevalence is not well documented. Many athletes with EIB or EILO may also experience BPD. The development of BPD in athletes is multi-factorial and likely to arise as a combination of poor posture, inappropriate activation of accessory respiratory muscles, incomplete expansion of rib cage and psychological factors (e. g. anxiety). Detection of BPD should include objective assessments and can be supported by appropriate questionnaires. Therapy for BPD can incorporate breathing pattern training, postural control, inspiratory muscle training and anxiety management. The therapy for BPD should be individualised as BPD can vary significantly between athletes.

Summary

- Athletes with BPD will not be able to complete high-intensity exercise sessions to the same extent as athletes without BPD.
- BPD can co-exist with other respiratory conditions e.g. asthma, EILO.

- Athletes can overcome BPD through individualised programmes that include education, breathing pattern retraining, IMT, anxiety management.
- Breathing pattern training should be progressed systematically from static supported postures through to function sport specific movements.
- Once BPD patterns have been overcome athletes should continue to engage in training 3–4 times a week to ensure they do not revert back to a dysfunctional pattern.

Multiple-choice questions

1. Athletes with BPD can have co-existing respiratory conditions such as asthma or exercise induced laryngeal obstruction.

   (A) True
   (B) False

2. When observing breathing pattern in an athlete and investigating for BPD you should look for ... (3 correct answers)

   (A) Chest but not abdomen movement
   (B) Accessory muscle activation
   (C) Blocked nose
   (D) Breath holding
   (E) Difficulty timing breathing with talking
   (F) Speed of speech

3. What musculoskeletal area do you not need to consider during BPD assessment?

   (A) Posture
   (B) Core stability
   (C) Pain
   (D) Muscle endurance
   (E) Spinal, thoracic and shoulder girdle mobility
   (F) Spinal and thoracic structure
   (G) Muscle strength, length and tension

4. Which is of the following methods cannot provide objective measurements of breathing pattern?

   (A) Opto-electronic plethysmography
   (B) Structured light plethysmography
   (C) Mouth Inspiratory Pressure
   (D) Brompton BPAT
   (E) Nijmegen questionnaire

5. The development of BPD in athletes is likely to arise through a combination ... (there are four correct answers)

(A) Poor posture
(B) Inappropriate activation of accessory respiratory muscles
(C) Weak inspiratory muscles
(D) Incomplete expansion of rib cage
(E) psychological factors (e.g. anxiety).

Key reading

Boudling, R., Stacey, R., Niven, R., Fowler, S.J. 2016. Dysfunctional breathing: a review of the literature and proposal for classification. *European Respiratory Review*. 25 (141) 287–294. Available at: http://err.ersjournals.com/content/25/141/287 [Accessed: 12 May 2018]

Bradcliff. 2018. Nijmegen questionnaire. Available at: www.bradcliff.com/for-the-client/questionnaire [Accessed: 5 May 2018]

Bradley, D. 2014. Physiotherapy in rehabilitation of breathing pattern disorder. In: *Recognising and Treating Breathing Disorders: A Multidisciplinary Approach*. London: Elsevier, 185–195.

Bradley, H., Esformes, J. 2014. *Breathing Pattern Disorders and Functional Movement International Journal of Sports Physical Therapy* 9 (1): 28–29. Available at: www.ncbi.nlm.nih.gov/pmc/a rticles/PMC3924606.

Bradley, D., Clifton Smith, T. 2005. *Breathe, Stretch and Move*. New York: Random House.

Burton, A., Lee, A., Yardley, L.et al. 2018. Physiotherapy breathing retraining for asthma: a randomised controlled trial. *The Lancet*. 6 (1): 19–28. Available at: www.thelancet.com/journals/lanres/article/PIIS2213-2600(17)30474–30475/fulltext [Accessed: 5 May 2018]

Buteyko Breathing Centre.,2018. Buteyko theory. Available at: www.buteyko.co.uk/buteyko-theory.htm [Accessed: 13 May 2018]

Chaitow, L., Bradley, D., Gilbert, C. 2014. The structure and function of breathing. In: *Recognising and Treating Breathing Disorders. A Multidisciplinary Approach*. London: Elsevier, 23–41.

Depiazzi, J., Everard, M.L. 2016. Dysfunctional breathing and reaching one's physiological limit as causes of exercise induced dyspnoea. *Breathe*. 12 (2): 120–129. Available at: www.ncbi.nlm.nih.gov/pmc/articles/PMC4933621/.

Dickinson, J., McConnell, A., Ross, E., Brown, P., Hull, J. 2015. The BASES Expert Statement on Assessment and Management of Non-asthma Related Breathing Problems in Athletes. *The Sports and Exercise Scientist*. 45. Available at: www.bases.org.uk/write/Documents/TSES_AUTUMN_2015_P8-9_(PAGES).pdf

Kroenke, K., Spitzer, R.L., Williams, J.B. 2001. The PHQ-9: Validity of a brief depression severity measure. *Journal of General Internal Medicine*. 16 (9): 606–613. Available at: www.ncbi.nlm.nih.gov/pmc/articles/PMC1495268 [Accessed: 10 September 2018]

McConnell, A. 2011. *Breathe strong*, perform better. Human Kinetics, U.S.A

Spitzer, R.L., Kroenke, K., Williams, J.B.W.et al. 2006. The GAD-7. *The Journal of Internal Medicine*. 166 (10): 1092–1097. Available at: https://jamanetwork.com/journals/jama internalmedicine/fullarticle/410326 [Accessed: 10 September 2018]

Todd, S.J., Livingston, R., Grillo, L., Menzies-Gow, A., Hull, J. 2016. Is the Brompton BPAT a useful tool to assess breathing pattern disorder in asthma? *Thorax*, 71 (3).

van Dixhoorn, J., Folgering, H. 2015. The Nijmegen Questionnaire and dysfunctional breathing. *ERJ Open Res.* 1 (1). Available at: www.ncbi.nlm.nih.gov/pmc/articles/PMC5005127/ [Accessed: 5 May 2018]

Answers: 1 (A), 2 (B,D,E), 3 (D), 4 (C), 5 (A,B,D,E)

12

ROLE OF RESPIRATORY MUSCLE TRAINING TO TREAT EXERCISE RESPIRATORY SYMPTOMS

Hege Havstad Clemm and John W. Dickinson

Overview

This chapter will cover:

- Indications for when respiratory muscle training (RMT) may be appropriate to use with athletes.
- Provide an overview of why athletes may benefit from RMT.
- Discuss how to conduct RMT.
- Why and when RMT is useful for athletes with breathing pattern disorders.
- Why and when RMT is useful for athletes with exercise induced laryngeal obstruction.

Introduction

As exercise intensity increases athletes will transition from predominantly nose to mouth breathing. In doing so, this alters the pattern of airflow in the upper airways as well as the relative distribution of resistance within the airway tree. When ventilation increases with increasing exercising intensity, a sense of dyspnoea may develop, if the athlete is unable to adapt their breathing pattern appropriately to this scenario (see Chapter 11). Furthermore, inadequate breathing patterns during exercise may lead to the development of laryngeal obstruction during exercise (see Chapter 9). All this will cause imbalance between air supply and air demand, leading to suboptimal conditions for gas exchange. As discussed in Chapter 11, efficient breathing patterns during exercise can to a certain extent be trained; with guidance in posture and head position, breathing frequency and depth, relaxation in the shoulder girdle and diaphragmatic breathing rather than clavicular breathing.

Some athletes find incorporating respiratory muscle training into breathing pattern training programmes to provide added benefit. As with other muscles in the body, the respiratory muscles can also be trained, for both strength and endurance. Respiratory muscle training (RMT) has been used in both health and disease to strengthen the diaphragm and other inspiratory muscles to enhance breathing efficiency. The theoretical basis behind the use of RMT is to make respiratory muscles work harder by forced breathing against an added resistance. The purpose is to make spontaneous breathing without this extra resistance feeling easier, thus improving function and performance. However, even if this concept is accepted, RMT should only be viewed as a supplemetary therapy for a variety of breathing disorders, and we still lack the proper guidelines for when to use this technique, in what patients and on which indications. For many athletes, both healthy and those struggling with breathing disorders like exercise induced asthma, exercise induced laryngeal obstruction (EILO) or breathing pattern disorder (BPD), RMT may prove to add value if used in the correct way.

What is the most beneficial form of RMT?

RMT is theoretically used to improve respiratory muscle strength, breathing quality, reduce dyspnea and off-set respiratory fatigue. Although it is possible to train both inspiratory and expiratory phases of the breathing cycle, previous research has demonstrated little benefit of utilising expiratory muscle training. Whereas, inspiratory muscle training has been shown to be of benefit to patients and athletes. There are several RMT-devises available on the commercial market using different principles, but no evidence based guidelines exist for what modality or which training program to use for different situations. We usually split RMT into two training modalities; strength and endurance. RMT devises can provide three types of breathing resistance: Flow resistive, pressure threshold and voluntary isocapnic hyperpnoea (the latter only for endurance training). The training program for RMT is in most cases set by the inspiratory resistance, calculated from a percentage of the maximum inspiratory pressure measurement (PImax or SIndex) the person is able to generate. The intensity of the training program is then dependent on breathing frequency and endurance; number of repetitions per day and number of weeks.

The most common outcome measurement for training improvement is maximum mouth inspiratory pressure (PImax), and most studies demonstrate significant improvement after training with RMT. The clinical benefit of an improvement in PImax is on the other hand not established and there exists no agreement on a threshold for clinically meaningful change in inspiratory strength or endurance. Results from several studies show only weak to moderate correlations between improvement in PImax and clinically meaningful measures like exercise tolerance, dyspnea and quality of life. The benefit of increasing PImax is therefore uncertain. However, a RCT study on 14 rowers showed a significant training effect associated with PImax, and even if VO_2 max and dyspnoea did not differ between the groups, those who had trained with RMT had significantly greater improvement in the 5000m trial time after 11 weeks. In some athletes, increases in PImax from RMT may have an additional effect on exercise performance. Two systematic reviews recently did a meta-analysis to evaluate the effect of RMT on healthy individuals and athletes. Training with RMT had a positive effect in general and the greatest effect on endurance performance in less fit individuals and in sports with longer durations. There was no improvement in exercise capacity among athletes, but the perceived breathlessness and exertion did improve after training with RMT. PI_{max} and maximal voluntary ventilation (MVV) improved among the athletes after both threshold training and isocapnic hyperpnoea training. In some athletes and in some sports, RMT also seemed to improve performance.

There is no consensus on when to use RMT and there is no scientific evidence supporting the routine use of RMT in athletes in general. The reason why some athletes seem to have an effect and some don't still remains uncertain.

HOW TO PERFORM RMT USING PRESSURE LOADED DEVICES

1. Ensure athlete has an appropriate breathing pattern (see Chapter 11).
2. Measure maximal inspiratory mouth pressure (PImax):

   a Athlete places device in mouth and passively expires to residual volume (RV).
   b Athlete instructed to inhale from residual volume to total lung capacity (TLC), utilising appropriate breathing pattern, with maximal effort.
   c This should be a rapid inspiratory breath but should be complete.

3. Set RMT device to appropriate resistance (see Table 12.1).
4. RMT training:

   a Athlete exhales slowly from TLC to RV, taking at least 5 seconds to reach RV, followed by a rapid inspiratory breath to TLC.
   b If athlete fails to reach TLC it may be a sign of fatigue or inappropriate breathing pattern.
   c During exhalation athlete should be encouraged to maintain good posture but relax any tension around thoracic region, shoulders and neck.
   d Repeat as per number of desired breathes for either strength or endurance (see Table 12.1).

How can I use RMT to retrain breathing pattern disorder (BPD)?

As discussed in Chapter 11, breathing pattern training can be helpful in resolving BPD in athletes. RMT can be incorporated within a breathing pattern training programme and it should not be used in isolation. As with other forms of strength training, movement pattern is a key component. Therefore, if athletes have inappropriate breathing patterns while engaging in RMT, this will likely act to reinforce the poor breathing pattern. Therefore, in athletes with suspected BPD, athletes must first modify their breathing pattern appropriately prior to engaging with RMT (see Chapter 11 for breathing pattern re-training). Once athletes have

TABLE 12.1 RMT training intensities

RMT intensity (% PImax)	Number of breathes	Target condition	Training focus
40–50%	30	Healthy athlete	Improve respiratory muscle strength
25–40%	30	Dysfunctional Breathing	Breathing technique
30–50% POWERbreathe	30	EILO	Improve opening of the larynx
(40)60–80% Respifit	Strength: 5 × 3 Endurance: 10–16 × 3		

demonstrated they are able to perform an appropriate inspiratory manoeuvre, utilising diaphragmatic breathing, they should be encouraged to start RMT.

When initiating RMT with athletes engaged in a breathing retraining programme, it is appropriate to initially train at a relatively low resistance (25–40%) of PImax. Using a lower pressure than recommended for improving respiratory muscle strength is appropriate for athletes with BPD, as it provides a greater opportunity for the athlete to execute appropriate breathing pattern. Once the athlete can easily complete the desired number of breathes, they should be encouraged to gradually increase the RMT resistance.

Digital RMT devices that enable to the athlete to gain immediate breath by breath feedback on the quality of their training can be of further benefit. These devices allow athletes to track power, air-flow and volume through each inspiratory manoeuvre. This allows the athlete to see if each breath achieved a smooth maximal breath. Figure 12.1 demonstrates the power production through the breath when athletes produce optimal and sub-optimal manoeuvres. It is clear when athletes utilise apical or asynchronic breathing patterns (see Chapter 11) they are unable to sustain power throughout inspiration and the total air inspired per breath is compromised. Allowing athletes to observe this detail provides immediate bio-feedback, which allows them to grasp what optimal breathing technique is. Regardless of the device it may assist athletes to have a practitioner place hands on sides of lower cage to allow them to focus on where they should initiate the breath. Alternatively, an elastic strap or band can be placed around lower rib cage – this should not provide extra resistance to work against.

As athletes improve and RMT becomes relatively easy standing still (Figure 12.2) they should be encouraged to conduct functional movement specific to their sport (Figures 12.3 and 12.4). Conducting functional RMT has been shown to have greater benefits for athletes when compare to static RMT. Examples of sports specific exercise are suggested in Chapter 11 and can also be found in a resource specifically dedicated to RMT for athletes.

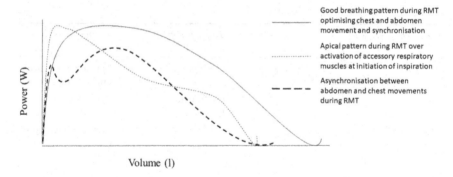

FIGURE 12.1 Power during RMT in optimal and suboptimal breathing patterns.

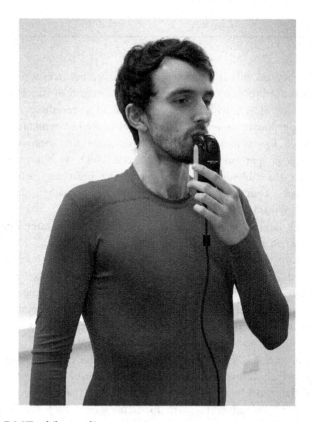

FIGURE 12.2 RMT while standing.

What is the theoretical basis for RMT as treatment for EILO?

The focus on RMT has often been on the diaphragm and accessory muscles and to increase maximal inspiratory (mouth) pressure (PImax) and/or maximal voluntary ventilation (MVV). A common way of thinking has been that RMT strengthens

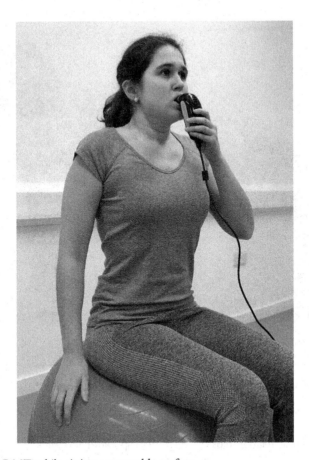

FIGURE 12.3 RMT while sitting on unstable surface.

the inspiratory muscles and patients that experience EILO would then be less likely to develop dyspnea and therefore delay the sense of panic. Some practitioners believe that in cases of persistent EILO, increased inspiratory strength may enable the person to generate sufficient pressure to overcome the laryngeal obstruction. However, then you risk exercising with ongoing stridor which may be harmful. Especially in the most common cases of EILO (i.e. with a tendency towards supraglottic closure), generating higher pressure trying to overcome the laryngeal obstruction may do more harm than good. When an athlete suffers from EILO, it is therefore recommended that the athlete focuses on on how to increase and strengthen the opening of the laryngeal inlet during exercise. Fatigue of the main abductor in the larynx, PCA muscle, has been suggested as a possible underlying pathology in one type of EILO. Rather than focusing on strength, appropriate breathing techniques and working with endurance and coordination in the larynx would perhaps be more beneficial. If we use RMT wisely, we can take advantage of the respiratory movement of the laryngeal inlet which is closely coordinated with the diaphragm.

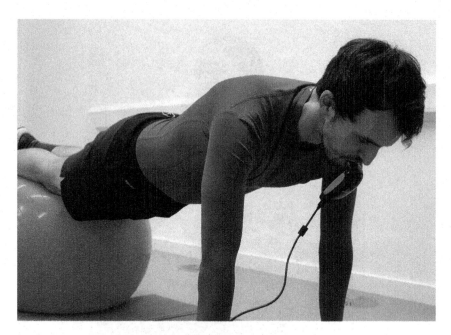

FIGURE 12.4 RMT while performing functional exercise.

WHY COULD RMT BE BENEFICIAL FOR EILO?

We take advantage of:

1. The phasic relationships between the diaphragm and the PCA-muscle. The PCA-muscle opens the laryngeal inlet slightly before contraction of the diaphragm.
2. The opening cascade in the larynx activated by pronounced inspiration.

RMT if utilised in the correct way may act to:

1. A more effective and better controlled laryngeal abduction.
2. Better coordination of the opening.
3. Reduced fatigue in the larynx.
4. More beneficial breathing pattern.

There are three case reports on direct use of RMT to increase the laryngeal areal. The reports include patients with persistent decreased glottal area and with vocal fold paralysis. All three patients reported decreased dyspnoea during exercise and speech after training with RTM. This indicates that one can use RMT to train the opening of the glottis directly.

Compared with the case reports on RMT increasing the laryngeal areal, those suffering from EILO have most often a normal larynx at rest, and the problem of obstruction is of a more dynamic character. The effect wanted from RMT is not just increased strength and widening of the larynx, but also coordination and better control. There is one study on 20 healthy subjects that investigated normal larynx response to RMT using a laryngoscope. This study showed that there are diverse laryngeal response patterns, underlining the complexity of the larynx. The results showed that 18 individuals opened their larynx when the PImax resistance was reduced to 60–80% compared with 10 at 80%. This study indicated that moderate resistance may be more beneficial to open the larynx than higher resistance. Reducing PImax may be more important when it comes to EILO training, also because it helps focus more on coordination.

Studies proving that RMT affects EILO are scarce. There are four case reports using RMT to treat EILO, which contain four patients with good effect and one with worsening. The reason why some subjects don't achieve a positive effect from RMT is a matter of investigation.

A recent publication on 30 athletes with EILO treated with RMT also demonstrated some diversity. This study reported a significant effect of RMT and suggests that RMT could be an efficient tool in conservative treatment of EILO, particularly in patients with a high degree of glottic obstruction. However, two of the athletes got worse from RMT treatment, so we need to be aware and individualise the approach to treatment and follow up. EILO is a heterogenic condition, with obstruction on either the glottis or supraglottic level or both. Different outcomes are illustrated by two subjects with similar symptoms, both of which were given RMT; one had a full recovery and the other got worse and needed surgery, most likely because of supraglottic stretching of the tissue due to the Bernoulli Effect. It is important to notice; when it comes to EILO, despite the heterogeneous findings, the symptoms are similar and you should always consider doing a continuous laryngoscopy during exercise test (CLE-test) before and to evaluate treatment effect. Because EILO is a heterogeneous condition that also may coexist with asthma, we always recommend doing a proper examination for both EILO and EIB before you start training with RMT.

What are the treatment principles of RMT for EILO?

The evidence so far points towards lower resistance, and endurance training rather than diaphragm strength and high resistance (PImax). We want maximal opening of the larynx, reduced fatigue of the larynx, and strengthening of the only abductor of the larynx and focus on coordination. However, it may depend on the larynx, the type of response you have and the type of EILO. Muscle strength training and neural adaptations need time. The neural pathways involved in new tasks are complex. At least 4 weeks are needed. However, this is still a field of investigation.

The first principle of treating EILO patients is to inform them that people may make many different noises and sounds when they become exhausted. When they make noise, they close the inlet and the airflow is obstructed. The first lesson is to try to breathe without any noise, to give the best airflow dynamics.

Second is the posture. Think of the respiratory tract as a tube; if you bend it, it will get a kink and the airflow will be obstructed. Try to hold your head high, keep your shoulders low and retracted.

Third is to learn how to use your breathing muscles correctly; use your thorax, widen it and relax in your throat, neck and shoulder girdle. Try to focus on breathing out from your belly and let the air stream in. This is called diaphragm breathing. Don't drag the air in through your throat; it will probably just have the effect of closing your larynx. This type of breathing can also be done rapidly. Focus on holding the larynx open while breathing, however it will make you dizzy, and using 'voluntary isocapnic hyperpnea' for this training can avoid dizziness.

When you are training with RMT and are breathing in against resistance, similar principles should be used. Widen your thorax, and use your diaphragm. Don't force the air in trough your throat and don't use clavicular breathing, your shoulders should be low and relaxed.

Breathing principles for keeping larynx open during exercise:

1. Don't make any breathing noises when breathing in.
2. Keep your head high and shoulders low.
3. Breath with your diaphragm – focus on exhalation and let the air stream in.

To resolve an attack of laryngeal obstruction:

1. Keep calm – try to avoid increased breathing rate.
2. Forced inspiration will only increase the problem – focus on exhalation.
3. Sniffing/breathing in through the nose.
4. Put your tongue behind the incisors during inhalation.
5. Try to yawn and breathe through it.

EXAMPLES OF RMT TRAINING PROGRAMS FOR EILO

1. Measure Maximal Mouth Inspiratory Pressure (PImax).
2. Two different training programs according to (a) POWERBreathe (Gaiam Ltd, Southam UK) or (b) Respifit (Biegler GmbH, Mauerbach, Austria):

   a Set the resistance on the training device to 40–60% of your maximum PImax Use an inspiratory muscle trainer and inhale 30 loaded breaths twice daily using the diaphragm and minimise cranial shoulder movements. Use 5 days per week.

   b Set the resistance on the training device to 60–80% of your maximum PImax

   • Day 1: Strength training with 5 maximal deep diaphragmatic inhalations repeated three times, separated by a one-minute break.

- Day 2 and 3: Endurance training: 12–16 slow/normal deep breaths for one minute repeated three times, separated with a 30 second break.

3.   Continue this cycle every day.
4.   Duration at least 6 weeks

Note: Regardless of training method it is essential that appropriate breathing pattern is utilised throughout (see Chapter 11).

CASE STUDY: EILO SUCCESSFULLY TREATED WITH SUPERVISED RMT

We here present an eighteen-year-old athlete struggling with breathing problems during exercise for many years. His symptoms were thought to be asthma, however difficult to treat. He had stopped competing due to his problem. There were no sign of asthma and examination with continuous laryngoscopy during maximal cardiorespiratory treadmill exercise (CLE) was used to visualise laryngeal movements from rest to peak intensity. EILO with supraglottic obstruction preceding glottic obstruction, become more pronounced with increasing respiratory demands. He was given a thorough physician-guided review of the video-recordings, structured breathing advice and reassurance. In addition RMT was given for 8 weeks. RMT consisted on training each day; strength training on 80% of maximum 1/3 of the time, and endurance training for 1 minute, 3 times, 2/3 of the time.

At follow-up after RMT he was content and reported better respiratory control. He had restarted training, aiming to resume competing. The second CLE-test revealed an open larynx with no adduction, neither glottic nor supraglottic. Peak oxygen consumption had increased by 10%. EILO can be successfully treated with RMT in many cases; it gives more control of the inlet and reduces fatigue. Unfortunately, not all patients treated with IMT are this successful and uncritical use of IMT in EILO can in some cases do more harm than benefit.

Conclusion

Breathing difficulties associated with exercise can to some extent be improved by re-training breathing pattern, and RMT can be a useful adjunctive tool in this regard. For some athletes RMT can help improve sports performance and it can reduce the experience of dyspnea and breathing fatigue and increase the MVV. However, the response to RMT is not uniform. RMT can be incorporated to the management of athletes with exercise induced bronchoconstriction, dysfunctional breathing and EILO. However, RMT should not be used in isolation and if delivered incorrectly can actually exacerbate breathing problems. RMT intensity can be modified to suit the training requirements of the athletes. In many cases more load is not a good thing as increasing RMT load may promote inadequate breathing technique. Athletes should focus on diaphragmatic breathing, keeping the training resistance under 80% of your PImax and a training ratio of 2:3 endurance versus strength. Using RMT appropriately may improve athletes breathing and sports performance. However, further research required to set standardised guidelines.

Summary

- RMT may be beneficial for athletes who experience BPD or EILO.
- Effectively undertaking RMT will condition upper (neck) and lower (chest and abdomen) respiratory muscles.
- RMT can focus on developing endurance or strength of the respiratory muscles. Training can be individualised for athletes to provide specific focus on the athletes particular respiratory issue.
- Optimising breathing pattern while performing RMT is essential to help athletes overcome EILO or BPD.
- Visual feedback during RMT can help an athlete develop an effective breathing pattern.

Multiple-choice questions

1. Which training modalities can we use for RMT?

    (A) Strength
    (B) Endurance
    (C) Both

2. What is of most importance when you are training opening of the larynx?

    (A) Strength
    (B) Endurance
    (C) Both

3. Which target condition need the lowest resistance?

    (A) EILO
    (B) Dysfunctional breathing
    (C) Healthy athletes

4. To abrupt an EILO attack – what is of most importance?

    (A) Try to get as much air in as possible
    (B) Increase the respirator rate
    (C) Keep clam and focus on exhalation

5. How long do you need to use the RMT to start to feel the effects?

    (A)   <4 weeks

    (B)   4–6 weeks

    (C)   >6 weeks

Key reading

Baker SE, Sapienza CM, Martin D, Davenport S, Hoffman-Ruddy B, Woodson G. Inspiratory pressure threshold training for upper airway limitation: a case of bilateral abductor vocal fold paralysis. *Journal of Voice*. 2003;17(3):384–394.

Clemm HSH, Sandnes A, Vollsaeter M, Hilland M, Heimdal JH, Roksund OD, et al. The heterogeneity of exercise induced laryngeal obstruction. *American Journal of Respiratory and Critical Care Medicine*. 2018; 197:1068–1069.

Dickinson J, Whyte G, McConnell A. Inspiratory muscle training: a simple cost-effective treatment for inspiratory stridor. *British Journal of Sports Medicine*. 2007;41(10):694–695.

Griffiths LA, McConnell AK. The influence of inspiratory and expiratory muscle training upon rowing performance. *European Journal of Applied Physiology*. 2007;99 (5):457–466.

HajGhanbari B, Yamabayashi C, Buna TR, Coelho JD, Freedman KD, Morton TA, et al. Effects of respiratory muscle training on performance in athletes: a systematic review with meta-analyses. *Journal of Strength and Conditioning Research*. 2013;27(6):1643–1663.

Illi SK, Held U, Frank I, Spengler CM. Effect of respiratory muscle training on exercise performance in healthy individuals: a systematic review and meta-analysis. *Sports Medicine*. 2012;42(8):707–724.

Mathers-Schmidt BA, Brilla LR. Inspiratory muscle training in exercise-induced paradoxical vocal fold motion. *Journal of Voice*. 2005;19(4):635–644.

McConnell A. *Breath Strong, Perform Better*. Champaign, IL: Human Kinetics; 2011.

Sandnes A, Andersen T, Hilland M, Ellingsen TA, Halvorsen T, Heimdal JH, et al. Laryngeal movements during inspiratory muscle training in healthy subjects. *Journal of Voice*. 2013;27(4):448–453.

Tong TK, McConnell AK, Lin H, Nie J, Zhang H, Wang J. 'Functional' inspiratory and core muscle training enhances running performance and economy. *Journal of Strength and Conditioning Research*. 2016;30(10):2942–2951.

Volianitis S, McConnell AK, Koutedakis Y, McNaughton L, Backx K, Jones DA. Inspiratory muscle training improves rowing performance. *Medicine and Science in Sports and Exercise*. 2001;33(5):803–809.

Answers: 1 (C), 2 (B), 3 (B), 4 (C), 5 (B)

13

EPILOGUE

Bringing it all together to optimise athlete respiratory care

John W. Dickinson, Jon Greenwell and James H. Hull

Overview

This chapter will cover:

- An approach to the delivery of an overall programme to optimise respiratory health in athletes.
- The place of screening or case detection and the benefits and pitfalls of this process.
- Screening tools that can be used to detect respiratory problems.
- The delivery and planning of a respiratory screening programme.
- Important aspects of how to present results and a subsequent treatment plan.

Introduction

Over the course of the previous chapters in this book, contributors have outlined the complex and often vexing respiratory issues that athletes and their support staff may face. It is clear from these chapters, that the assessment of respiratory problems such as cough, recurrent respiratory tract infection or nasal symptoms, in athletic individuals, is not always straightforward. In this unique population, symptoms often relate poorly to objective evidence of respiratory disease. Indeed, as discussed in Chapter 5, exercise respiratory symptoms in isolation are a poor predictor of the presence of exercise induced bronchospasm (EIB) in athletes and the symptoms athletes describe could, as easily, be caused by other conditions discussed elsewhere in this book, such as exercise induced laryngeal obstruction (EILO). Equally athletes may struggle with symptoms impacting their performance and yet to fail to recognise or report symptoms and therefore receive no investigation or further support.

Inadequate management of respiratory issues can lead to sub-optimal training, performance and general wellbeing. It is thus vital that any clinician or allied professional who is involved, either directly or indirectly, in the care of an athlete should (a) have an understanding of the implications and impact of respiratory problems and (b) have a system in place to try and detect and effectively manage these problems.

The aim of this chapter is thus to pull together a number of the issues described in the preceding chapters and share our experience, over many years, of supporting athletes with respiratory issues; from the position and viewpoint of respiratory consultant, team medical officer and respiratory physiologist/therapist. In this chapter we will discuss various activities and procedures that can help facilitate optimal care and ongoing support for your athletes.

Should you screen athletes for respiratory issues?

The first step in appreciating or detecting respiratory issues in athletes is to acknowledge that they exist and indeed are prevalent. Thus, in a team of twenty endurance athletes, the published evidence suggests that somewhere between 3–5 members of that team will experience respiratory symptoms or indeed actually have EIB. It is also likely that a similar proportion or more have nasal or upper airway issues and that these issues often overlap in the same individual. Having acknowledged this fact, some may therefore argue that it is somewhat remiss of any team medical strategy, not to consider how you can correctly identify affected athletes and then optimise their care and thus their health and performance.

Some form of medical screening for athletes is now fairly commonplace and widely undertaken across most sports, especially in an elite context (e.g. professional football and cycling). Screening can be employed in various guises, but is advocated with the overall purpose and mandate of detecting reversible medical problems, with the ultimate aim that it is undertaken with the purpose of optimising health. Frequently cited examples of athlete screening programmes include cardiac screening to detect and prevent sudden cardiac death in athletes and musculoskeletal screening to try and reduce risk of injury. Indeed, several sports now mandate cardiac screening programmes (e.g. UEFA for young elite footballers). Currently, screening for respiratory problems is however not widely undertaken, despite the substantial evidence that previously undiagnosed EIB is common in high level athletes.

The general concepts of screening, as a process, are as applicable when applied to the context of athlete health as they are to any other medical condition. Specifically, for a screening programme to be effective there are a number of key characteristics that should be assessed and satisfied (Table 13.1). For example, it is important that the precision and performance of any screening tool is known before it is applied, so as not to cause unwanted distress due to misdiagnosis. Likewise, although it might seem immediately obvious and logical to look for any possible condition that might impact performance, this has to weighed against the risk of false-positive diagnosis and for example the implications and time taken out by a squad to undergoing testing.

A further consideration is that in its purest sense, screening is used to detect a condition that might otherwise remain completely occult/hidden (e.g. to detect cardiac problems in athletes). This therefore differs from circumstances in which you might preferentially select a cohort of athletes, struggling with respiratory symptoms or recurrent infection. Often the latter is more appropriately classified as *case detection* or *case confirmation* and in fact may be a more targeted and thus an appropriate means of optimising care and overall team performance.

Adopting a screening policy for respiratory conditions in athletes may provide a solution to improve detection and management of upper and lower airway issues in athletes, proving the key screening characteristics are satisfied in the target population of interest (see Table 13.1). This strategy may improve the airway health of athletes and there is some emerging evidence in football (soccer) players that aerobic fitness may also partially improve. The application of such a programme may however not be appropriate in a population with a low background prevalence of respiratory problems (e.g. boxers). How you apply this approach thus very much depends upon the athletic population to whom it concerns, the resources available and your overall ability to action/make direct changes to an athlete's care, from the results that ensue.

TABLE 13.1 Criteria and considerations when screening athletes for exercise-induced bronchoconstriction

Criteria	Considerations
The condition – understood, important, and clearly defined	Significant literature. Defined; but debate and variable application of defining criteria.
Prevalence	Reasonably well known. Considerable differences between studies highlight potential difficulties with test result interpretation and application. Highest prevalence in endurance athletes.
The diagnosis – testing • Reasonable cut-off values • Good test-retest reliability	IOC-Medical Commission most relevant to elite athletes. EVH valid and reliable, but not widely available, and costly.
The overall policy • Cost effective • Valid and reliable • Safe	Facilities available in developed nations, but not worldwide. Currently no available data on cost effectiveness.
Effective treatment readily available	Optimum treatment debated. Potential negative effects of treatment.

What should a respiratory screening or case detection programme involve?

In 2004, we initiated a screening programme for Olympic athletes representing Team GB. This initially focused on the need to give a formal diagnosis of asthma or EIB to enable the athletes to obtain a therapeutic use exemption (TUE) under the WADA guidelines at the time. At this time, the testing mainly encompassed bronchoprovocation challenge and little else. Since then the process has evolved and over the past ten years the assessment process has expanded to consider assessments that could be considered more of a 'total airway approach'. i.e. addresses issues not only relating to potential asthma but also those impacting other sections of the respiratory system.

WHAT ASSESSMENTS CAN BE INCLUDED IN A RESPIRATORY SCREENING PROGRAMME?

- Take previous history and ask specifically whether athlete experiences any of the following during or after exercise:

  - coughing
  - wheezing on breathing in or breathing out
  - excess mucus production
  - difficulty in breathing in or breathing out
  - dizziness
  - nausea

- Enquire whether symptoms worsen in any of the following environments:

  - hot or cold weather
  - low or high humidity
  - dusty
  - high pollen and/or exposure to known allergies
  - high pollution

- Consider using questionnaires to detect EILO (Newcastle LHQ and Pittsburgh VCD), allergy (AQUA) and ENT (RQLQ, SNOT-22) issues
- Baseline maximal measures of:

  - FeNO
  - flow-volume loops
  - peak inspiratory nasal flow

- Bronchodilation challenge (if baseline FEV_1 <80% predicted value and airflow obstruction, i.e. generally taken as $FEV_1/FVC<0.7$)
- Bronchoprovocation challenge (if baseline FEV_1 ≥80% predicted value); include reversibility challenge if challenge is positive.

What is the value of including validated questionnaires in respiratory screening?

Several questionnaires can be used to detect problems in the respiratory tract. Unfortunately the only questionnaire validated in athletes is the Allergy Questionnaire for Athletes (AQUA). It is therefore necessary to be cautious when interpreting questionnaires such as the Rhinoconjuctivits Quality of Life Questionnaire (RQLQ), the Sino-nasal outcome test 22 (SNOT-22) and the Asthma Quality of Life Questionnaire (AQLQ) or Asthma Control Questionnaire (ACQ). This being said the results from these questionnaires should still be useful in terms of highlighting problems and informing more targeted clinical focus on a specific area.

There are a number of questionnaires that can look at laryngeal symptoms. These include the Newcastle Laryngeal Hypersensitivity Questionnaire (Newcastle LHQ) and the Pittsburgh Vocal Cord Dysfunction (Pittsburgh VCD) questionnaire. A positive score on these questionnaires will not be enough alone to give a definitive diagnosis of EILO, but may lead the clinician undertaking the screening to look more closely at laryngeal irritability, whether that be due to reflux, EILO, dysfunctional breathing or medication side effects, particularly from dry powder inhalers.

Finally, gastro oesophageal reflux as a possible underlying cause of cough or stridor can be assessed using the Hull Airways Reflux Questionnaire (HARQ).

Using objective respiratory screening investigations – what is best?

The choice of bronchoprovocation challenge is often determined from a synergy between pragmatic limitations and the logistical capabilities of a given screening session. Although an exercise challenge is the logical choice because of its ecological value, in practice it is often difficult to standardise, and field-based tests in particular run the risk of delivering a sub optimal minute ventilation. In addition, if the exercise challenge is field-based, it is difficult to account for the environment on the day of the assessment. i.e. the weather may be relatively warm and humid and an athlete report's problems in the cold and dry. Accordingly, when evaluating athletes with mild EIB, you may need to consider undertaking multiple exercise challenges, on various days, due to the issues around test standardisation and environment.

A pragmatic approach is thus to incorporate a sensitive surrogate means of detecting EIB. In this context, we have utilised EVH testing and found this to be the most practical provocation test to deliver. However, when an EVH challenge is not possible a Mannitol challenge (i.e. an indirect bronchoprovocation test) can be used. The delivery and interpretation of bronchoprovocation testing is covered in depth in Chapter 5, but in keeping with the approach to any form of medical test, clinicians should be cognisant of the limitations of the test in the context of a given clinical scenario; i.e. just because a EVH test demonstrated a 12% fall in FEV_1 post challenge (i.e. mild positive), this doesn't automatically imply that the athlete's symptoms are solely arising from EIB.

An additional advantage of an EVH test, or a static exercise test, such as cycle ergometer, over a field-based test or a methacholine challenge, is it allows an assessment of the breathing technique to be made if the person undertaking the test has experience in this. Specifically, this allows the clinician to detect sub-optimal breathing patterns (see Chapter 11 for more detail), which can exist either in the presence of a positive or negative test for EIB. It is not unusual to see a multiple diagnosis of EIB +/– EILO +/– dysfunctional breathing pattern, and it is always important to be aware that this may happen and to put in place a logical treatment plan for *all* conditions (see Chapters 6, 7 and 11).

Fraction of exhaled nitric oxide (FeNO) measurement is easy to perform with a handheld device, and in itself can be a simple and useful screen for the presence of airway inflammation. This can be difficult to interpret in athletes who are already established on or currently prescribed inhaled corticosteroid treatment but in a new case, it is useful in terms of informing treatment choices (i.e. a heightened level indicates a potential for inhaled steroid response). It also gives a baseline score that can be used to look at response, and potentially compliance with medication at repeat testing. i.e. to ensure that airway inflammation has been adequately controlled (Figure 13.1).

Finally, to ensure thorough airway assessment, it is vital to evaluate any sinonasal contribution from the upper airways as well, using nasal peak flow, as well as using screening questionnaires to look at possibly underlying allergy (see Chapter 8 for further detail). It is vital to treat recurrent allergy or nasal congestion in athletes, whether they be pool based or land based, as these are often the underlying cause of cough or upper respiratory tract infections. Again, overall a good screening programme should be able to detect multiple pathologies, and not just treat for EIB in isolation (see Figure 13.2).

What to do with the results of a respiratory detection programme?

Before a screening or detection programme is organised it is important to be clear as to who has the responsibility for giving the results to the athlete, their coach and their family if appropriate, in a timely manner. In addition, who is responsible for prescribing any new medication, making any changes to existing medication regimes and who is going to teach and/or check inhaler technique. From a clinical governance perspective, it should also be clear where the results will be stored.

If the screening takes place in a professional club, or national programme then the screening would usually be supervised by the club/team doctor, and the responsibility would be theirs. It is likely that the athlete's family doctor, or general practitioner in the United Kingdom will take on the long term prescribing of the medication. So the athlete's general practitioner should also be informed with a copy of the results, and a covering letter explaining why the screening took place, what the diagnosis is and clear documentation as to the medication that is to be used.

If an athlete has been diagnosed with EIB then time should be taken to explain what this means in terms of long term health implications (if any), potential side effects of any medication and benefits of treatment, particularly if this is a new diagnosis in a previously asymptomatic individual, and what the outcomes of not starting medication may be in the short or long term. The use of specific medications is covered in Chapter 6.

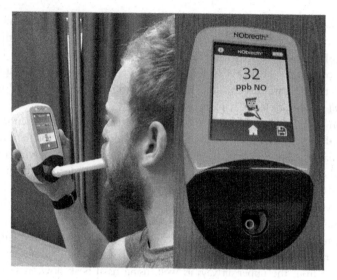

FIGURE 13.1 Measuring the fraction of exhaled nitric oxide.

MANAGING THE RESPIRATORY HEALTH OF THE 2016 OLYMPIC GREAT BRITISH SWIMMING TEAM

In the build-up to the 2016 summer Olympic Games members of Great British (GB) swimming team had their respiratory health and function assessed annually between 2014 and 2016.

Fifteen members of the Olympic team were confirmed to have EIB via a positive EVH challenge. Following the identification of EIB the swimmers were monitored to investigate the impact of the prescribed inhaler therapy in the lead up to the 2016 Olympic Games in Rio.

Three months prior to the Olympics, the swimmers had their respiratory health reviewed. This included spirometry, FeNO and a verbal assessment with a respiratory consultant. Inhaler technique was also assessed.

In the final respiratory review FeNO was significantly reduced (pre: 27.7 ± 15.1, post: 16.3 ± 6.5 ppb; $p = 0.006$), this change was more pronounced in those who initially had a FeNO above normal (> 25ppb) (pre: 40.7 ± 8.4, post: 19.4 ± 6.8 ppb, $p = 0.002$).

FEV_1 at rest was unchanged (pre: 4.8 ± 1.1, post 4.8 ± 1.1 L, $p = 0.775$). Three swimmers had airway obstruction at rest (FEV_1 < 80% predicted value). They were administered 200 mcg of Salbutamol, which improved FEV_1 above baseline by 12.9 ± 7.7%.

All swimmers had at least one coexisting condition alongside EIB; 63% reflux, 53% laryngeal closure, 68% nasal disease, 47% recurrent infection and 63% abnormal breathing sensations. Inhaler technique was good except for rate of inhalation; the recommended rate is 30 L.min^{-1}, whereas the swimmers inhaled at a rate of 344 ± 52 L.min^{-1}. 37% reported side effects from inhaler use. Inhaler therapy was altered where appropriate following these assessments.

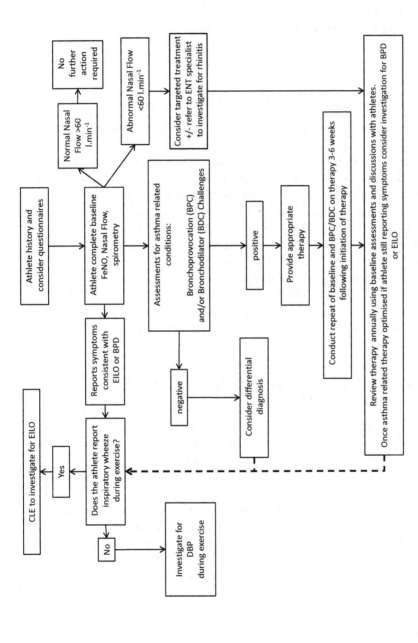

FIGURE 13.2 Algorithm for the assessment and management of respiratory health in athletes.

Notes: CLE, continuous laryngoscopy during exercise; DBP, Dysfunctional breathing pattern; EILO, Exercise induced laryngeal obstruction; ENT, Ear, nose and throat; FeNO, Fraction of exhaled nitric oxide.

Our work with the GB swimmers demonstrates that although EIB is a common issue in elite swimmers, the complete pulmonary system should be considered when attempting to optimise respiratory health. Respiratory health in elite swimmers can be optimised through regular assessment, treating the whole airway and individualising therapy management.

General considerations and opportunities at screening

The respiratory screening process also offers an opportunity to discuss illness prevention, particularly with respect to upper respiratory tract infection (e.g. infection avoidance and hand-washing), and also annual vaccination against the influenza virus.

In athletes with a previous diagnosis of EIB or asthma, an assessment of inhaler technique should be made, using a similar device to their usual inhaler. This should include spacer use and an assessment of good oral hygiene post inhaler administration. If appropriate this is a good opportunity to provide education on correct technique as a vast majority if athletes will have inhalation that is too aggressive limiting drug delivery to the lungs. This is also a good opportunity to discuss compliance with the existing medication regime, and work to improve this through education if required.

It is helpful to have all information in a written version, as there is often a lot of information to take to recall. At the same time written outcomes from the review should include appropriate contact details in case the athlete, their GP, or family have any subsequent questions.

DISCUSSING ANTI-DOPING IMPLICATIONS AND RESPIRATORY CARE

- The current WADA guidelines should be discussed (www.wada-ama.org/en/what-we-do/the-prohibited-list). There is often a misconception that a Therapeutic Use Exemption (TUE) form is needed for all asthma medication, by athletes and coaches. Only a few asthma medications actually currently require a TUE.
- The maximum allowed dosage dose of β_2-agonists within 12 and 24 hours need to be explained to the athlete to avoid any accidental adverse analytical findings.
- The website www.globaldro.com provides comprehensive up-to-date information and athletes and coaches should be advised to check any medication and its implications in sport, on this site.

When to involve a specialist?

There are certain scenarios when involvement of a broader multi-disciplinary team and specifically a respiratory or allergy specialist will be indicated. For example, in the case of suspected EILO, it may be necessary to arrange exercise laryngoscopic assessment (see Chapter 9). Despite the high prevalence of respiratory problems in athletes there is actually very few specialists who have expert knowledge in the care of athletes. International guideline documents provide guidance and many of the key clinicians and specialists globally are involved and contribute to these guidelines (i.e. these documents can serve as a guide to signpost potential contacts in your region).

If the athlete has been given a diagnosis of breathing dysfunction or EILO then again it should be clear who will be involved in co-ordinating the rehabilitation programme. This may include some or all of the wider sports medicine team; doctor, physiotherapist, nutritionist, sports psychologist and coach as well as specialist allied health professionals such as respiratory physiotherapists and speech and language therapists.

How should an athlete be monitored once treatment has been initiated?

Best practice dictates that patients with a new diagnosis of respiratory problems are regularly reviewed to ensure adherence with prescribed treatment, to assess the response to treatment both subjectively and objectively and evaluate any side effects/review understanding of the condition. Objective assessment could typically include baseline spirometry *on medication* if there was evidence of airflow obstruction at baseline testing and if not then a repeat provocation challenge +/− repeat FeNO testing. Inhaler technique should be re-checked regularly given there is generally poor recall of the steps of good inhaler use and thus inhaler errors often re-occur over time. If any exercises have been prescribed for EILO or dysfunctional breathing then the efficacy of these techniques should be assessed. Moreover, if an athlete with EILO has not improved then it would be appropriate to consider referral for direct laryngoscopy.

In our experience, at a repeat testing review, it is not unusual to encounter athletes, who previously didn't have any symptoms at the time of baseline testing, to now report improvement that was previously attributed to a 'lack of fitness'. If not and an athlete, repots no difference at all then a pragmatic conversation will be needed to discuss the ongoing importance of inhaler therapy, based upon the other investigation results and measures such as baseline lung function and airway inflammation.

In terms of longer-term follow-up, it is logical to consider annual surveillance of respiratory health in athletes with a known diagnosis and arrange a regular surveillance programme. An opportune time to review the treatment plan often falls at a pre- season or end of season screening/training camp.

EXAMPLE OF THE BENEFITS OF MONITORING IMPACT OF THERAPY FOLLOWING INITIAL SCREENING AND DETECTION OF EIB

Between 2017 and 2019 Olympic Games the GB swimming team adopted an annual review of athletes with respiratory issues. As part of this review athletes were identified with EIB via an EVH challenge where invited to complete a further EVH challenge a year later while using there prescribed therapy.

Nineteen elite competitive swimmers of the Great British swimming squad, competing regularly at international level participated in the review. Each athlete provided data on two screening visits, separated by a calendar year. On each visit, athletes completed baseline exhaled nitric oxide (FeNO) and EVH challenge. A positive EVH challenge ($EVH_{positive}$) was deemed if a swimmers FEV_1 fell ≥10% from baseline at two consecutive time points, with greatest fall defined as FEV_{1max}. Following first screening (EVH_1), $EVH_{positive}$ athletes were prescribed appropriate inhaler therapy in accordance to their FEV_{1max}. On the subsequent testing visit, $EVH_{positive}$ swimmers were asked to continue prescribed EIB therapy leading up to the repeated EVH challenge (EVH^2), to assess EIB control when actively using EIB therapy.

Swimmers were grouped depending on adherence to therapy. Non-adherent, hence completed two EVH challenges with no active medication ($EVH^1 \rightarrow EVH^2$; $n = 13$) and those who adhered to EIB therapy ($EVH_{OFF} \rightarrow EVH_{ON}$; $n = 6$).

Swimmers with EIB who used their prescribed inhaler therapy had a reduction saw a fall in the fall FEV_1 post EVH challenge the year after they initiated therapy (–9.17 ± –3.4%) when compared to the baseline assessment of therapy (–26.7 ± –13.3%; $p = 0.02$). The swimmers with EIB who did not continue to use their inhaler therapy one year after initiating therapy had a similar fall in FEV1 post EVH between the initial (–14.1 ± 3.9%) and follow-up (–13.3 ± 5.0%; $p = 0.148$).

Elite swimmers diagnosed with EIB and adherent to inhaler therapy, displayed greater protection to hyperpnoea induced bronchoconstriction than when not using therapy. Swimmers whom were non-adherent with EIB therapy demonstrated agreement with previous EVH challenge result. This case study highlights the importance for elite athletes with EIB to remain adherent with to inhaler therapy, as it helps preserve airway health. Furthermore, the inclusion of an EVH challenge during annual screening or case detection is effective at monitoring EIB control in elite swimmers.

CASE STUDY: A CYCLIST WITH A COUGH

When you start working with a new cycling team one of the riders comes to talk to you after a race. They tell you that whenever they need to make a hard effort in a race, they start to cough afterwards and feel that they can't catch their breath. Some of the riders have commented how they are quite noisy with their breathing. They feel that this is impacting on their performance.

When you ask about what they have been advised in the past they tell that they were given a Salbutamol inhaler and were told it was due to asthma, over time they've steadily started to increase the number of times they take it, sometimes 8–10 times a day. They feel that this has helped a bit with the cough, but not the breathlessness. On further questioning they tell you that their nose often feels blocked, for which they sometimes use a decongestant for a few days at a time, and that they can't drink some of the sports drinks that the team uses as it causes a burning in their throat. They have missed 6 days of racing due to viral infections this season, but aren't particularly worried as this is normal for them.

This is a typical example of what a sports medicine doctor can be presented with, a multitude of possible causes, but no testing or screening has taken place. A presumed diagnosis of asthma has been given, with limited treatment effect, but now there is a risk of exceeding the WADA maximum dosage.

The athlete in this case would be perfect for a holistic screening programme, looking at allergy, reflux, illness prevention, inhaler technique, testing for exercise induced bronchoconstriction and looking at breathing patterns. This may help to persuade the coaches of the team that other athletes, with seeming minor problems can benefit from screening, reduce time loss to illness and improve wellbeing in racing.

Are there any challenges in setting up respiratory screening in groups of athletes?

Sports physicians, respiratory medicine physicians and respiratory physiologists will often have conversations with coaches and administrators from different sports about the benefits of respiratory screening and there can be a difference of opinion. Generally, the response falls into one of three different groups:

1. Perfectly happy to screen all of the athletes in their group.
2. Agree to screen those athletes who they may see have a potential respiratory diagnosis, and coaches/team physio will often identify those that they would like to be screened.
3. Reluctant to allow any of their group to be screened.

The reluctance for screening can be due to a variety of factors including:

1. New diagnosis of EIB requires the use of medication to manage it. Leads to two issues:

     a   Treating a previously undiagnosed problem and they feel that we are unnecessarily using medication, particularly with the stigma in some sports, particularly cycling, of the use of salbutamol, and also of a 'steroid' inhaler, and that this is being used to enhance performance.

     b   Diagnosis may validate any illness and lead to increased time loss to training.

2.   Coaches struggle to identify time to fit in testing as it may result in losing training time.

3.   Coach feels athletes are reluctant to buy into testing as they may act negatively towards identification of a respiratory issue.

When introducing a respiratory screening programme it is useful to be prepared for these responses and to explain that the reason is solely to optimise athlete health and availability. There is some emerging evidence that the value of a screening programme is to improve athletic performance, both directly (i.e. by enhanced exercise ventilatory performance) and indirectly (i.e. by improved health leading to a reduced number of missed days due to respiratory illness).

Another misconception is that athletes either have a diagnosis of EIB, in which case they are treated, or that they do not have EIB and so do not have a respiratory problem, so no further intervention is required. Certainly, over the past few years, an improved understanding and appreciation of EILO and breathing pattern dysfunction (see Chapters 9 and 11) has helped many athletes receive appropriate treatment, even in the absence of EIB.

Other potential challenges include the practical implications and logistics of screening. A screening programme needs to be fitted around training, for example an exercise test or EVH test cannot be performed within 4 hours of finishing training, which invariably means the days training needs to be rearranged. Many athletes and coaches will be reluctant to alter even one days training, unless they can see a clear benefit in their performance. For athletes who have a historical diagnosis of asthma and are prescribed inhalers, due consideration needs to be given for the *wash-out* period of any inhaler medication (i.e. to ensure that testing doesn't reveal a false negative diagnosis). This almost always causes a degree of concern and needs to be addressed; it is especially valuable to test this group of athletes, as it is not unusual to come across an athlete with a historical diagnosis of asthma, who has a negative provocation test, and so a re-evaluation of their management is required, particularly if they still report symptoms. Moreover, the WADA guidance is quite clear that a diagnosis of asthma made in childhood is not sufficient proof that an adult has a diagnosis and thus if a therapeutic use exemption certificate (TUE) is required then confirmatory proof of the diagnosis is needed in an adult athlete.

BARRIERS OFTEN CITED TO ORGANISING A RESPIRATORY SCREENING PROGRAMME

- Only useful for those that have symptoms.
- Don't want to miss training to undertake the testing programme.

- Not necessary if you already have a diagnosis of asthma.
- Coaches or athletes not wanting to use medication as maybe seen to be performance enhancing if the athlete does not have a wheeze.
- Athlete doesn't want to take steroids, and misunderstanding as to what is in the inhaler.
- The diagnosis may validate any illness and lead to increased time loss to training.

LOGISTICS AND CONSIDERATIONS WHEN SETTING UP A SCREENING PROGRAMME

- Should always be a doctor on site in case of medical emergency.
- Access to salbutamol inhaler with spacer or alternatively a nebuliser.
- Ability to measure height and weight.
- Consent forms for athletes.
- Information sheets for athletes.
- Sterile environment so reusable mouthpieces/mask for EVH challenge can be cleaned.
- Ability to sterilise spirometer turbine.
- Safe storage and delivery process for EVH gases that meets national guidelines.
- Enough time built into screening timetable if part of a larger medical screening programme/day.
- Suitably trained staff to interpret spirometry to ensure that all lung function has returned to normal before athlete is safe to go home.

Summary

The overall aim of this book is to provide an overview of the way in which respiratory problems can affect athletes and how to detect and best treat them. In this final chapter we have summarised some of the key points to consider when planning an overall strategy to optimise respiratory health. We have addressed some of the common logistical issues and provided details on a pragmatic way to approach this area. Now it's over to you …

Key reading

Ansley, L., Rae, G. & Hull, J. H. (2013). Practical approach to exercise-induced broncho-constriction in athletes. *Prim Care Respir J*, 22(1), 122–125.

Bonini, M., Braido, F., Baiardini, I., Del Giacco, S., Gramiccioni, C., Manara, M., Taglia-pietra, G., Scardigno, A., Sargentini, V., Brozzi, M., Rasi, G. & Bonini, S. (2009).

AQUA: Allergy Questionnaire for Athletes. Development and validation. *Med Sci Sports Exerc*, 41(5), 1034–1041.

Dickinson, J. W., Whyte, G. P., McConnell, A. K. & Harries, M. G. (2005). Impact of changes in the IOC-MC asthma criteria: a British perspective. *Thorax*, 60(8), 629–632.

Hopkins, C. (2009). Patient reported outcome measures in rhinology. *Rhinology*, 47(1), 10–17.

Hull, J. H., Ansley, L., Garrod, R. & Dickinson, J. W. (2007). Exercise-induced broncho-constriction in athletes-should we screen? *Med Sci Sports Exerc*, 39(12), 2117–2124.

Jackson, A. R., Hull, J. H., Hopker, J. G. & Dickinson, J. W. (2018). Impact of detecting and treating exercise-induced bronchoconstriction in elite footballers. *ERJ Open Res*, 4(2). doi:10.1183/23120541.00122-2017.

Juniper, E. F. & Guyatt, G. H. (1991). Development and testing of a new measure of health status for clinical trials in rhinoconjunctivitis. *Clin Exper Allergy*, 21, 77–83.

Levai, I. K., Hull. J. H., Loosemore, M., Greenwell, J., Whyte, G. & Dickinson, J. W. (2016). Environmental influence on the prevalence and pattern of airway dysfunction in elite athletes. *Respirology*, 21(8), 1391–1396.

Morice, A., Spriggs, J. & Bell, A. (2011). Utility of the Hull airways reflux questionnaire in the assessment of patients in the acute admissions unit. *European Respiratory Journal*, 38, 3513.

Vertigan, A. E., Bone, S. L. & Gibson, P. G. (2014). Development and validation of the Newcastle laryngeal hypersensitivity questionnaire. *Cough*, 10, 1. doi:10.1186/1745-9974-10-1.

ACKNOWLEDGEMENTS

Dr Dickinson:

To all the teachers, coaches, scientists and medical practitioners I have had the pleasure to either learn from, work with, mentor or watch from afar, I thank you for being the foundation and illumination of my understanding of sports science, respiratory medicine and elite sport.

In particular, Dr. Mark Harries, Prof. Greg Whyte & Prof Alison McConnell. They had the foresight to improve the respiratory care that British Olympic athletes received. I am so grateful that in 2003 they let me loose on the British Olympic team in the preparation for the Athens 2004 Olympic Games. I will be forever appreciative of their knowledge, support and friendship.

To Rebecca, the awesome Joseph, the marvellous Emily and my wider family; thank you for your belief, fun and love. YNWA.

Dr Hull:

Special thanks to Rachel, my daughters Izzy and Chloe, and my wider family, for their support. Also, a special thanks to the physiology staff and my clinical colleagues at the Royal Brompton Hospital, London and to Prof. Mike Loosemore, ISEH, UCL for his support.

Both:

We would both like to thank all our world leading, wonderful, talented and knowledgeable author contributors. Thank you for providing your time, expertise and support for this project. Thank you to the Routledge publishing team for their support, advice, patience and expertise in designing and marketing the book. To all the incredible athletes we have worked with, you have been an inspiration. It has been a pleasure to support you and contribute, in a small way, to your successes.

INDEX